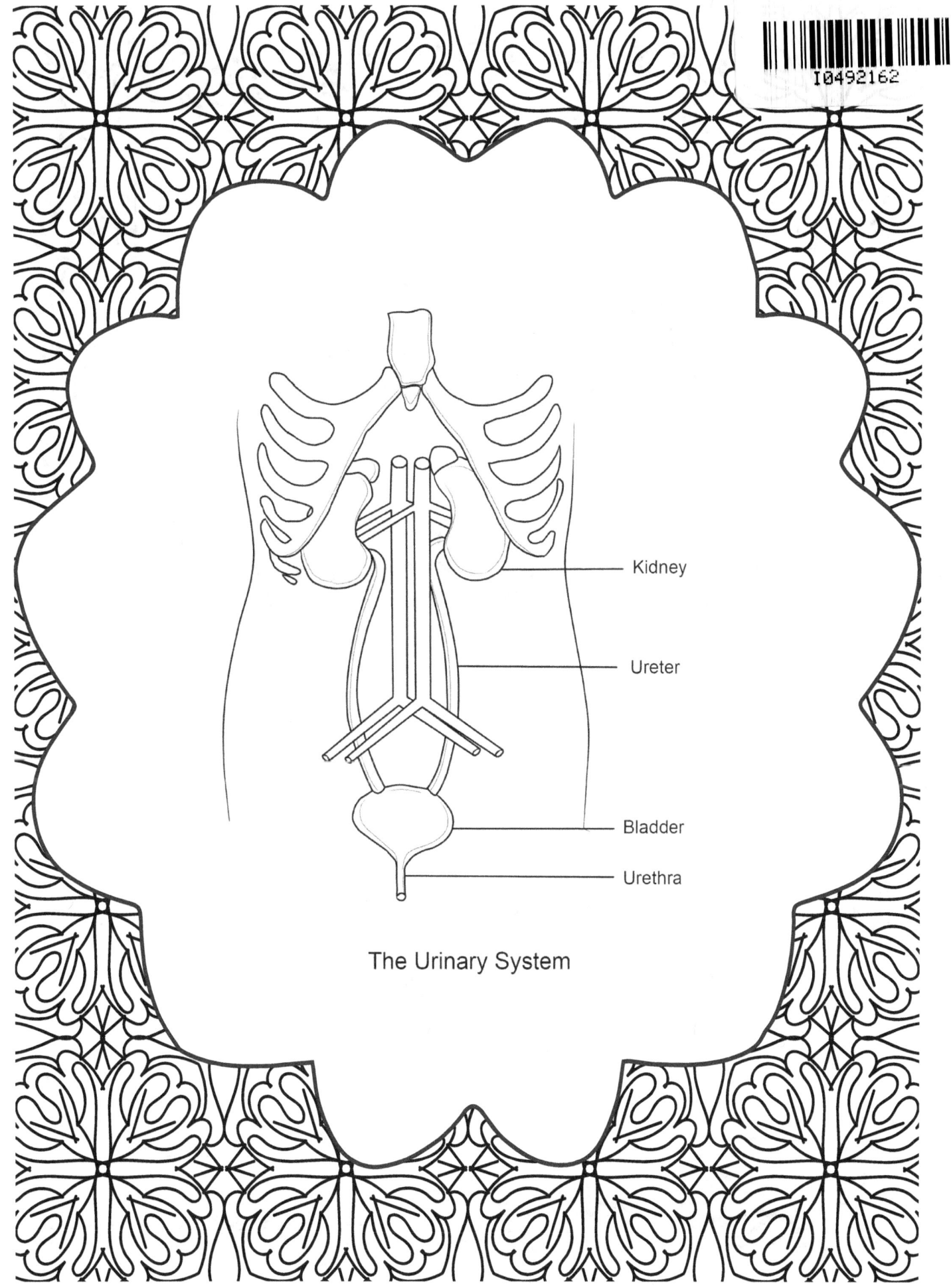

Kidney

Ureter

Bladder

Urethra

The Urinary System

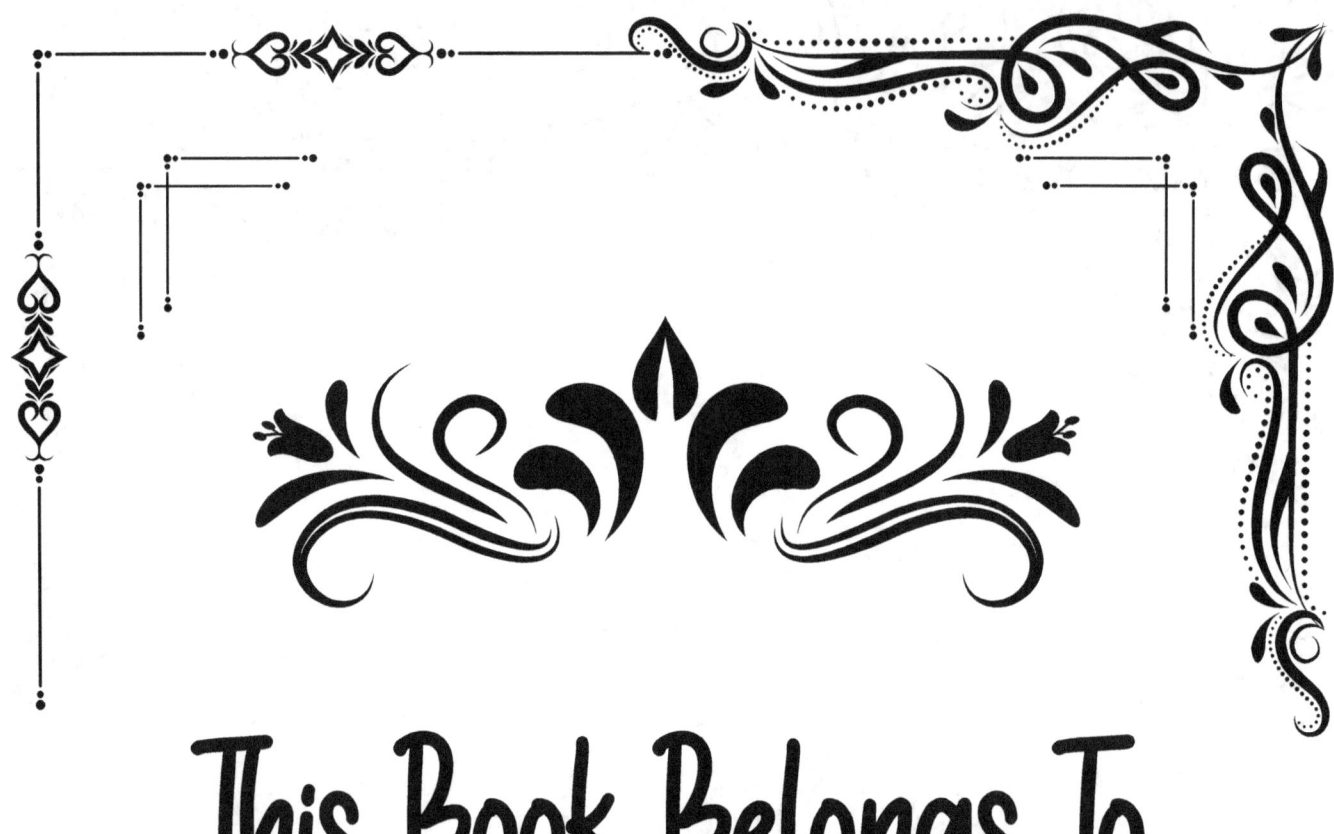

This Book Belongs To

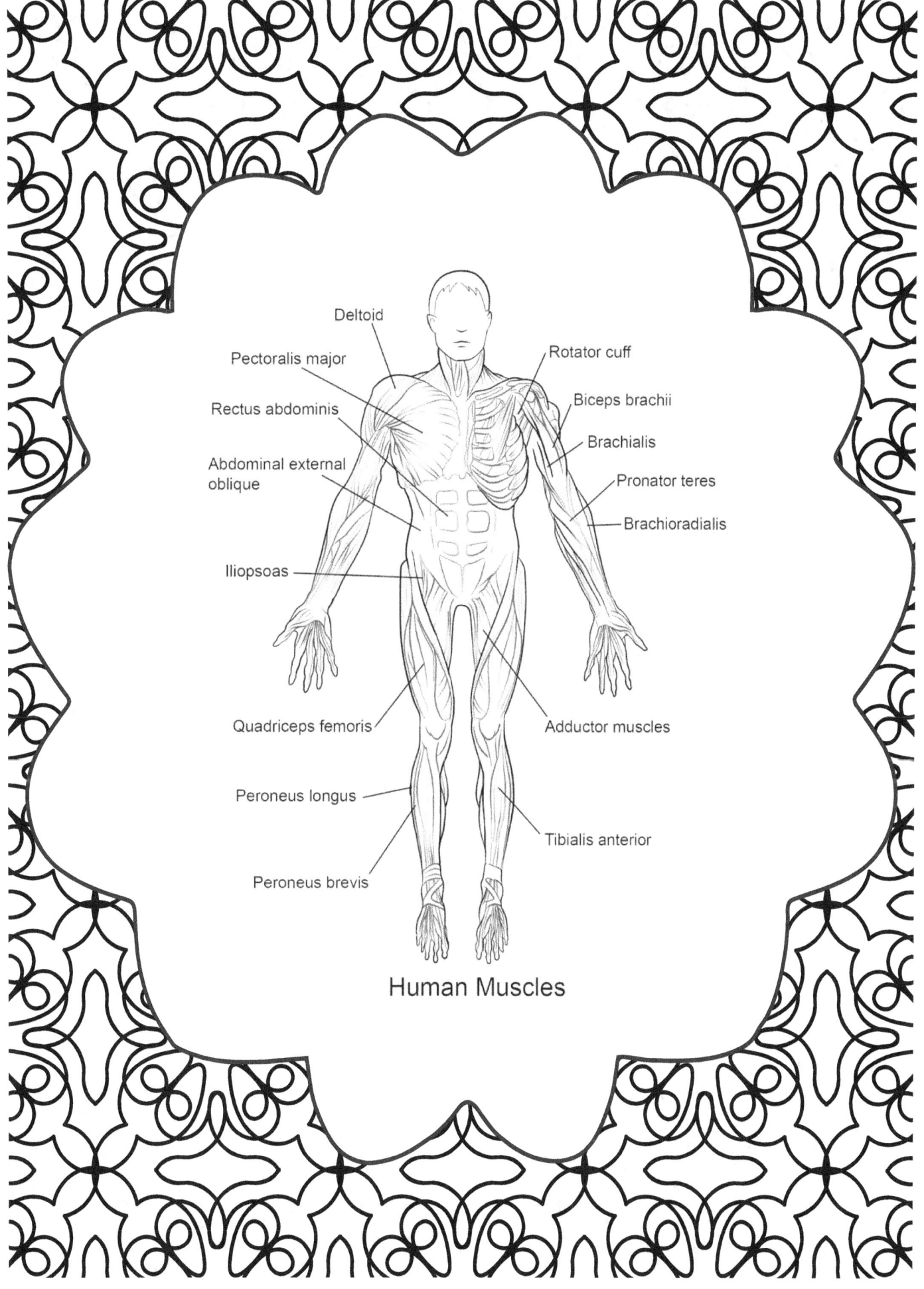

Deltoid

Pectoralis major

Rectus abdominis

Abdominal external
oblique

Iliopsoas

Quadriceps femoris

Peroneus longus

Peroneus brevis

Rotator cuff

Biceps brachii

Brachialis

Pronator teres

Brachioradialis

Adductor muscles

Tibialis anterior

Human Muscles

Gallbladder Anatomy

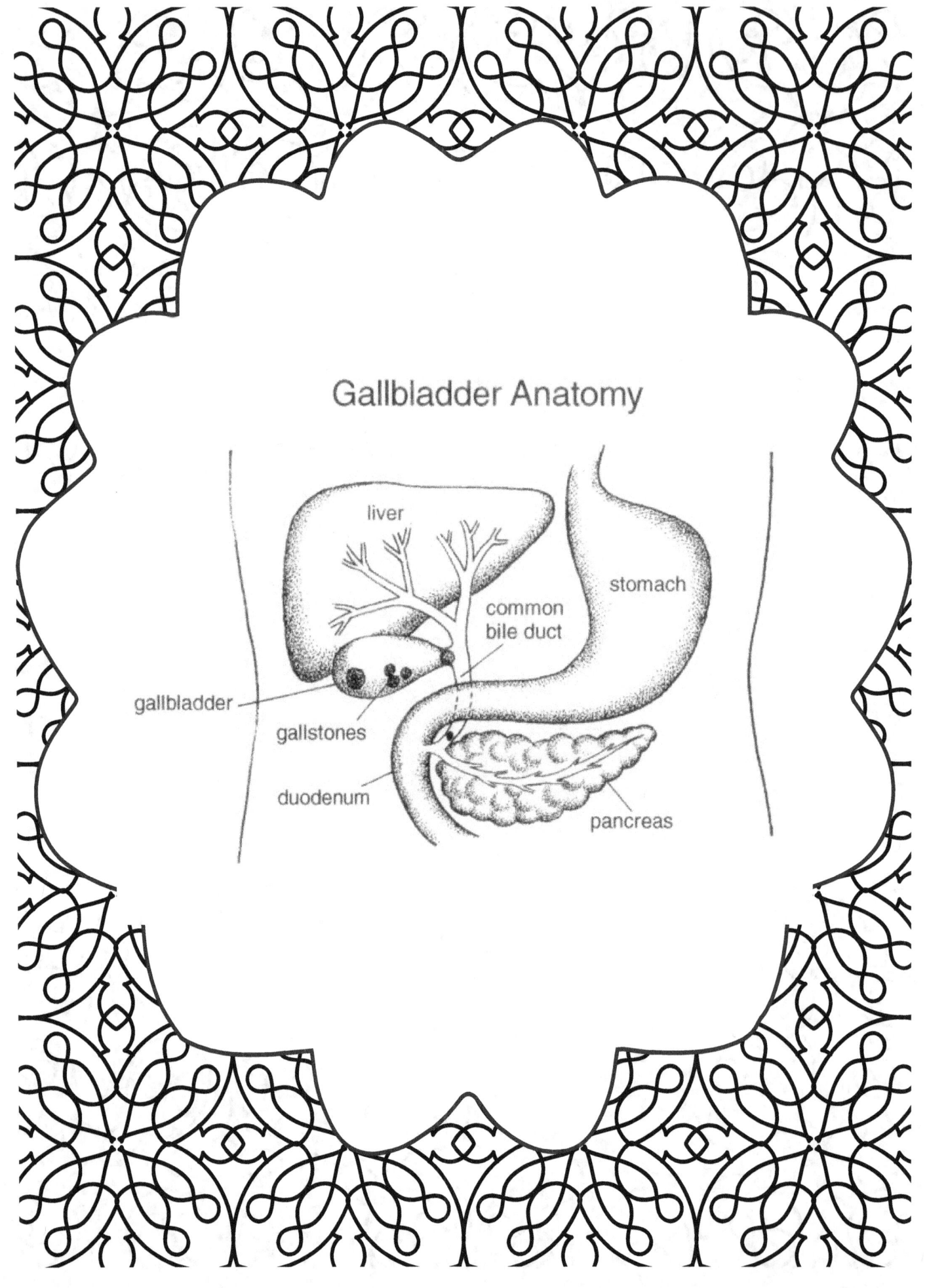

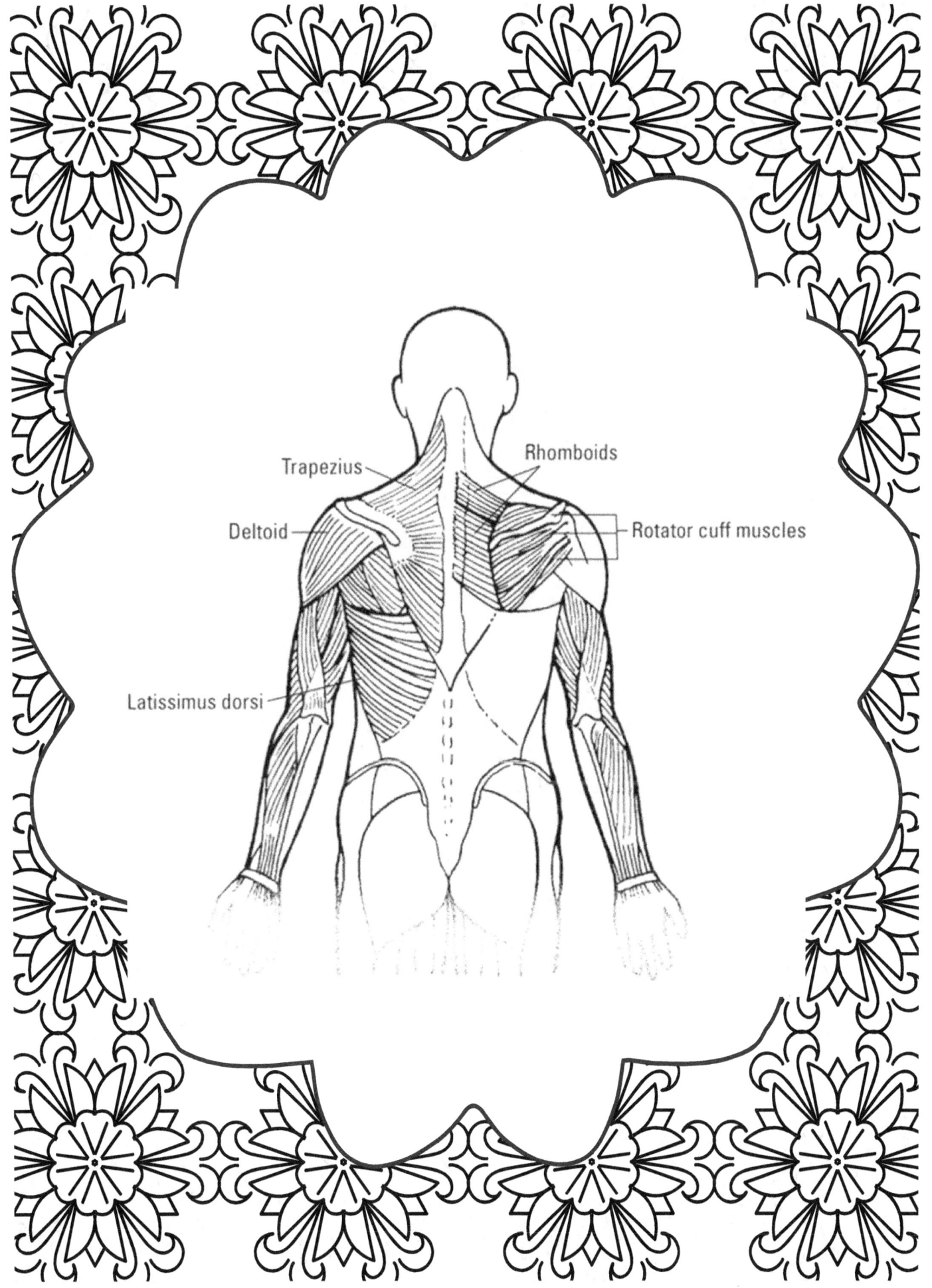

Trapezius

Rhomboids

Deltoid

Rotator cuff muscles

Latissimus dorsi

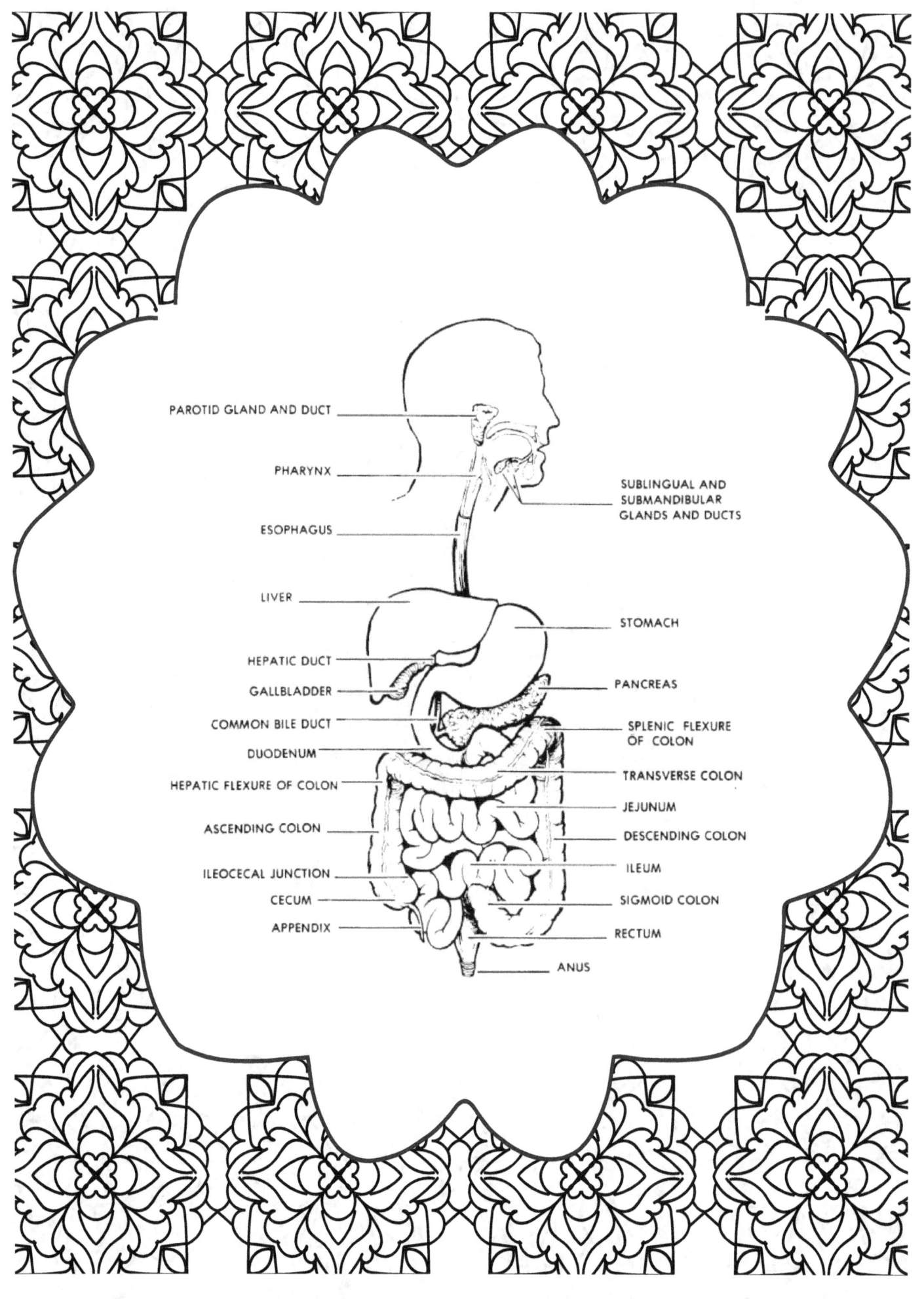

PAROTID GLAND AND DUCT

PHARYNX

ESOPHAGUS

SUBLINGUAL AND
SUBMANDIBULAR
GLANDS AND DUCTS

LIVER

STOMACH

HEPATIC DUCT

GALLBLADDER

PANCREAS

COMMON BILE DUCT

DUODENUM

SPLENIC FLEXURE
OF COLON

HEPATIC FLEXURE OF COLON

TRANSVERSE COLON

ASCENDING COLON

JEJUNUM

DESCENDING COLON

ILEOCECAL JUNCTION

ILEUM

CECUM

SIGMOID COLON

APPENDIX

RECTUM

ANUS

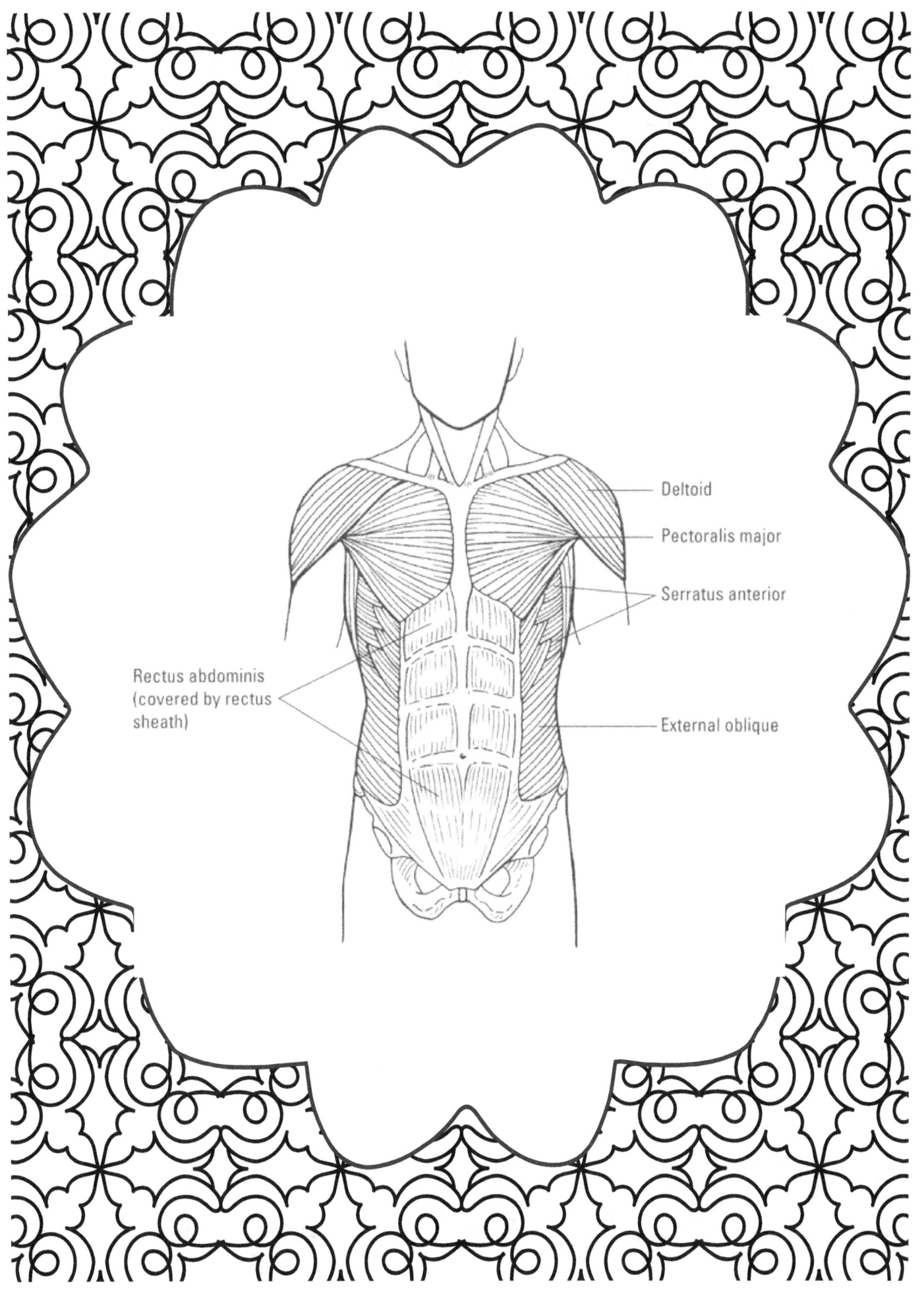

Deltoid

Pectoralis major

Serratus anterior

Rectus abdominis
(covered by rectus
sheath)

External oblique

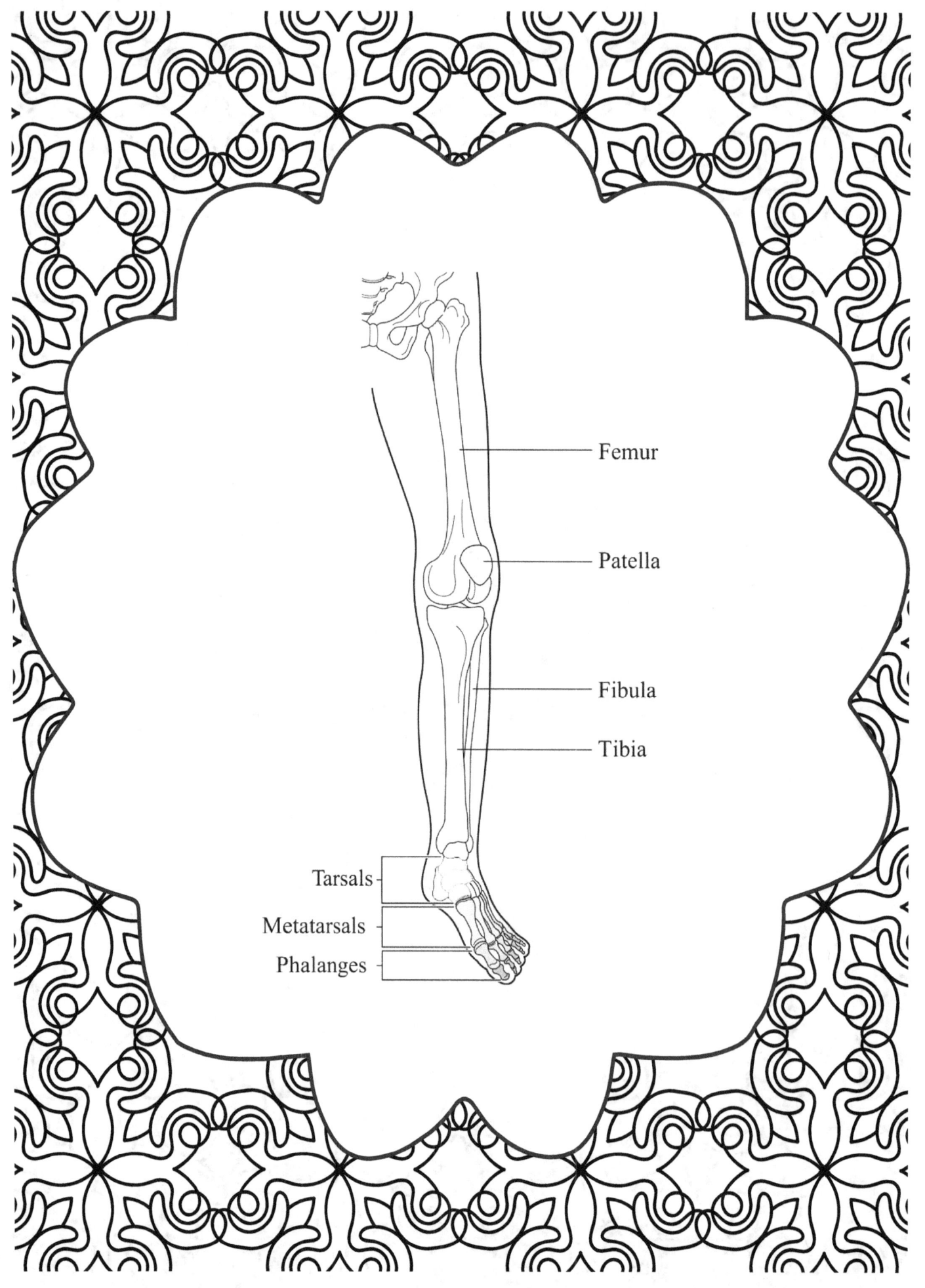

Femur

Patella

Fibula

Tibia

Tarsals

Metatarsals

Phalanges

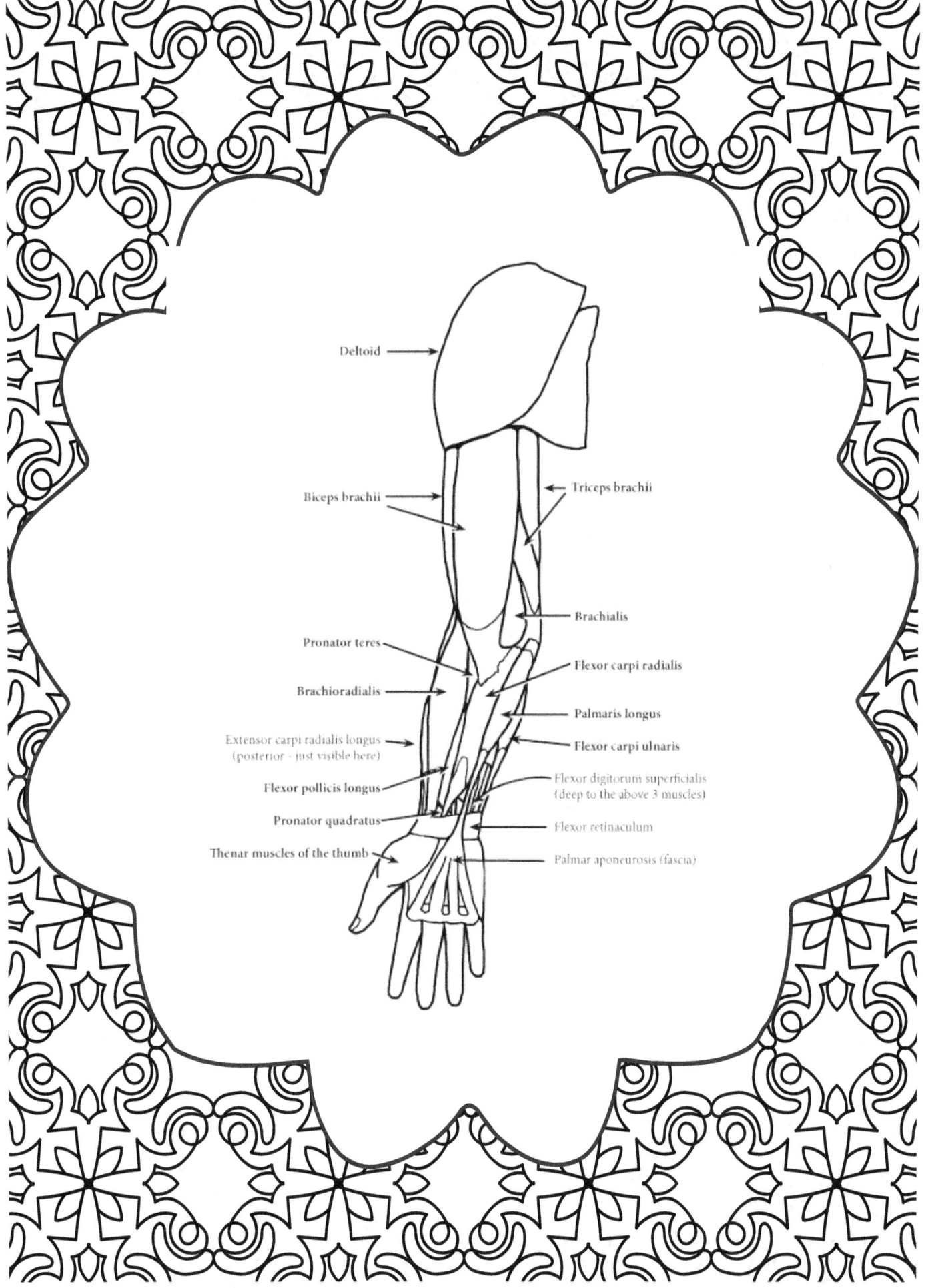

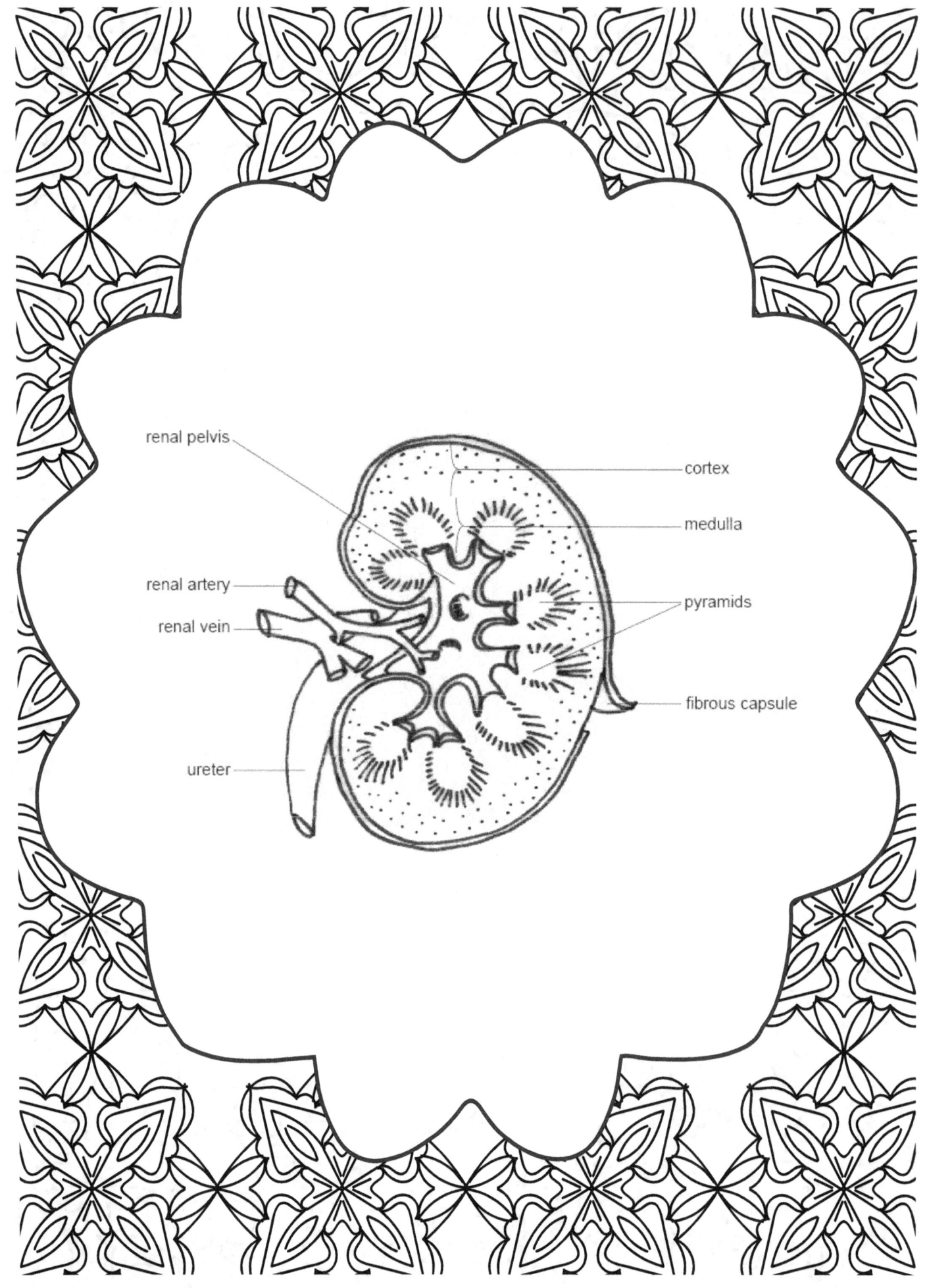

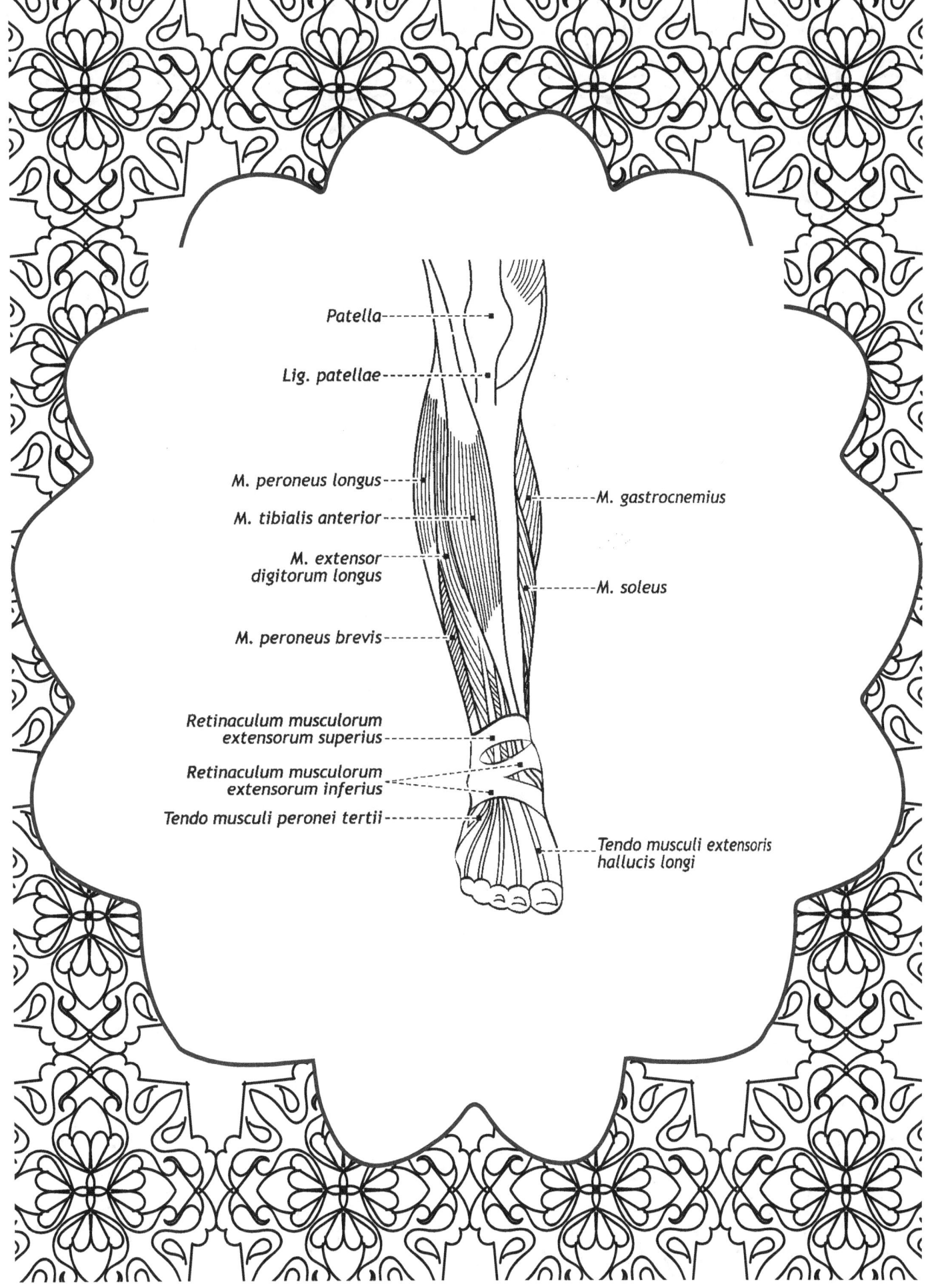

Patella

Lig. patellae

M. peroneus longus

M. tibialis anterior

M. extensor
digitorum longus

M. peroneus brevis

Retinaculum musculorum
extensorum superius

Retinaculum musculorum
extensorum inferius

Tendo musculi peronei tertii

M. gastrocnemius

M. soleus

Tendo musculi extensoris
hallucis longi

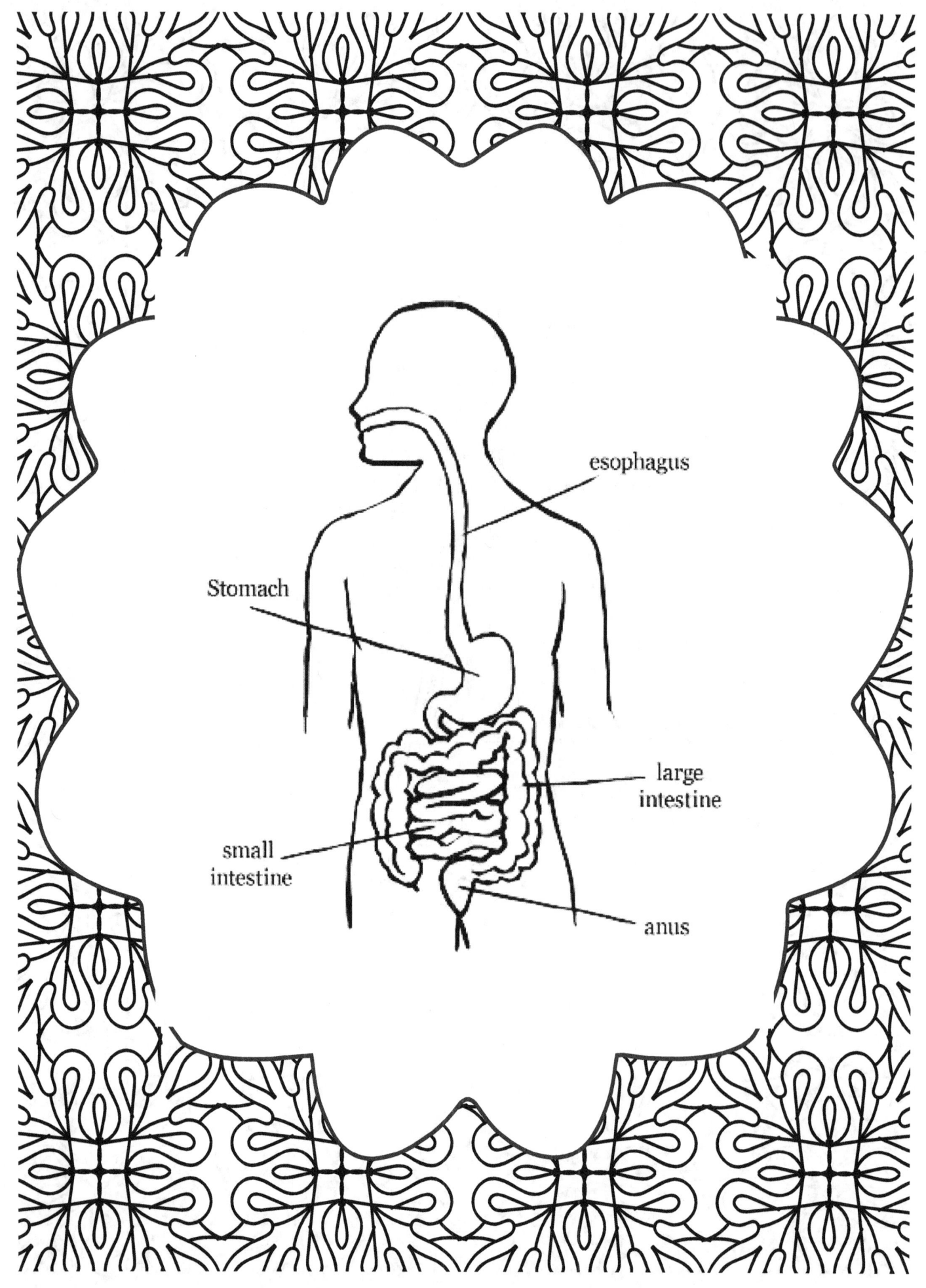

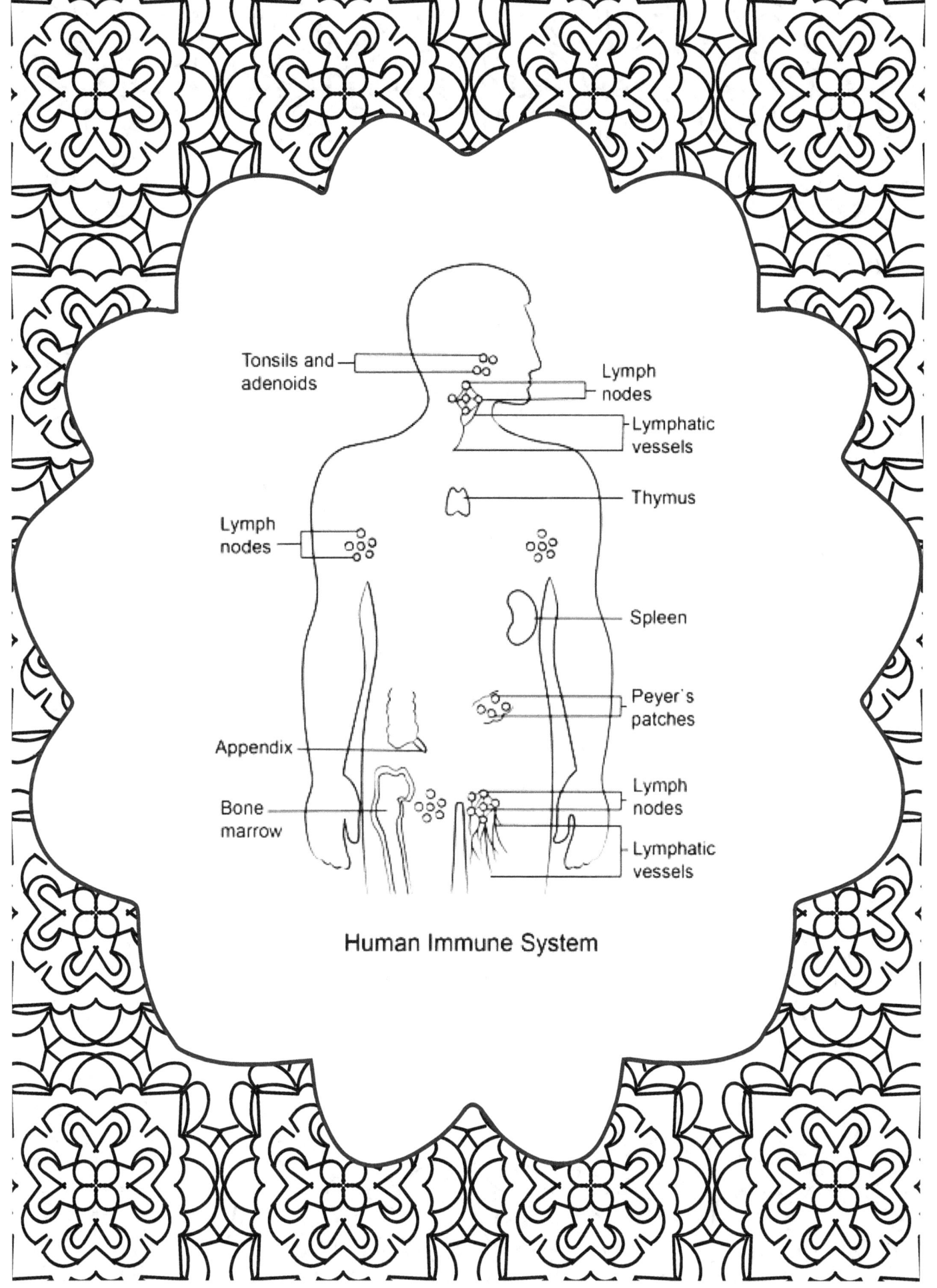

Human Immune System

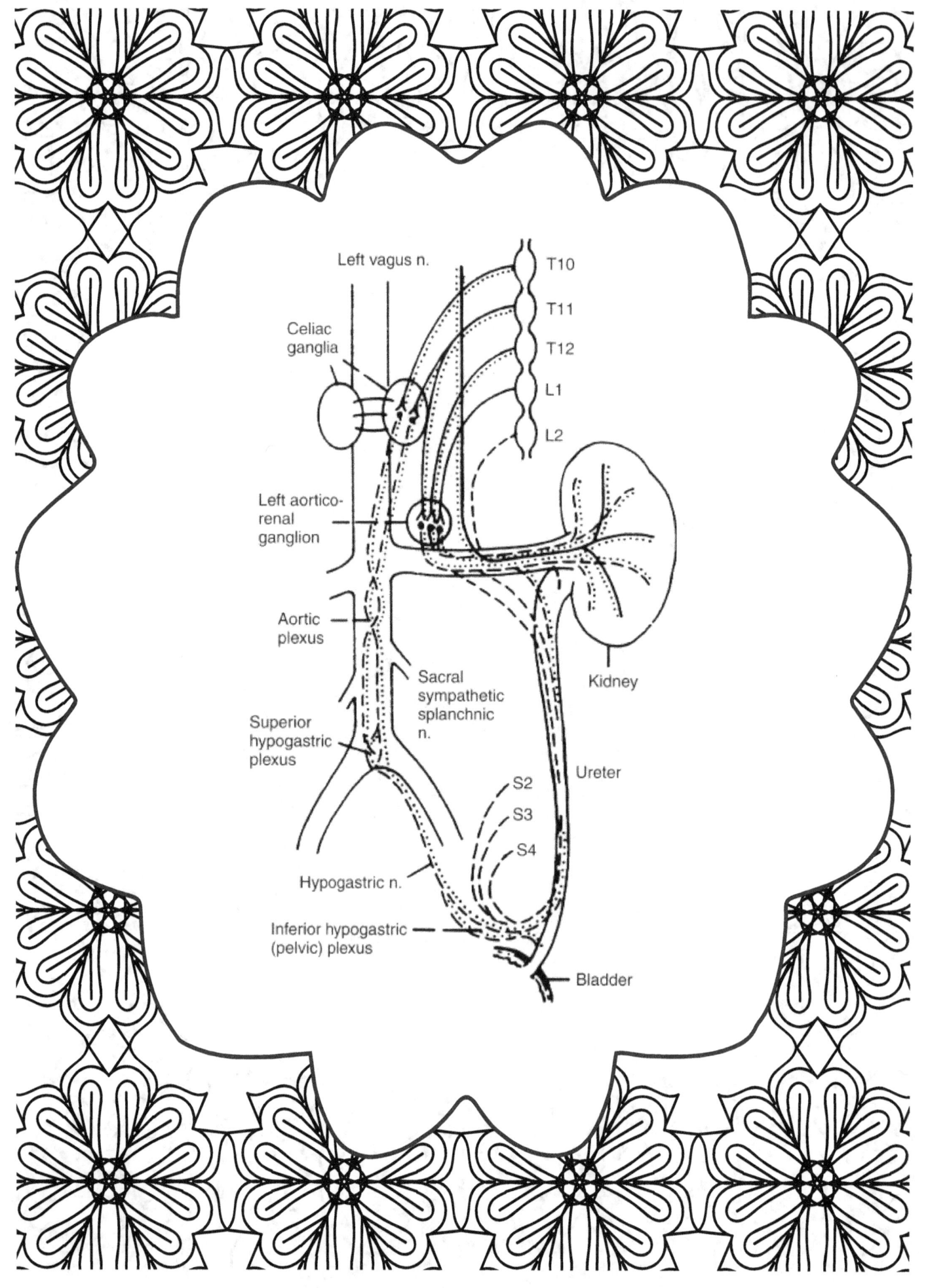

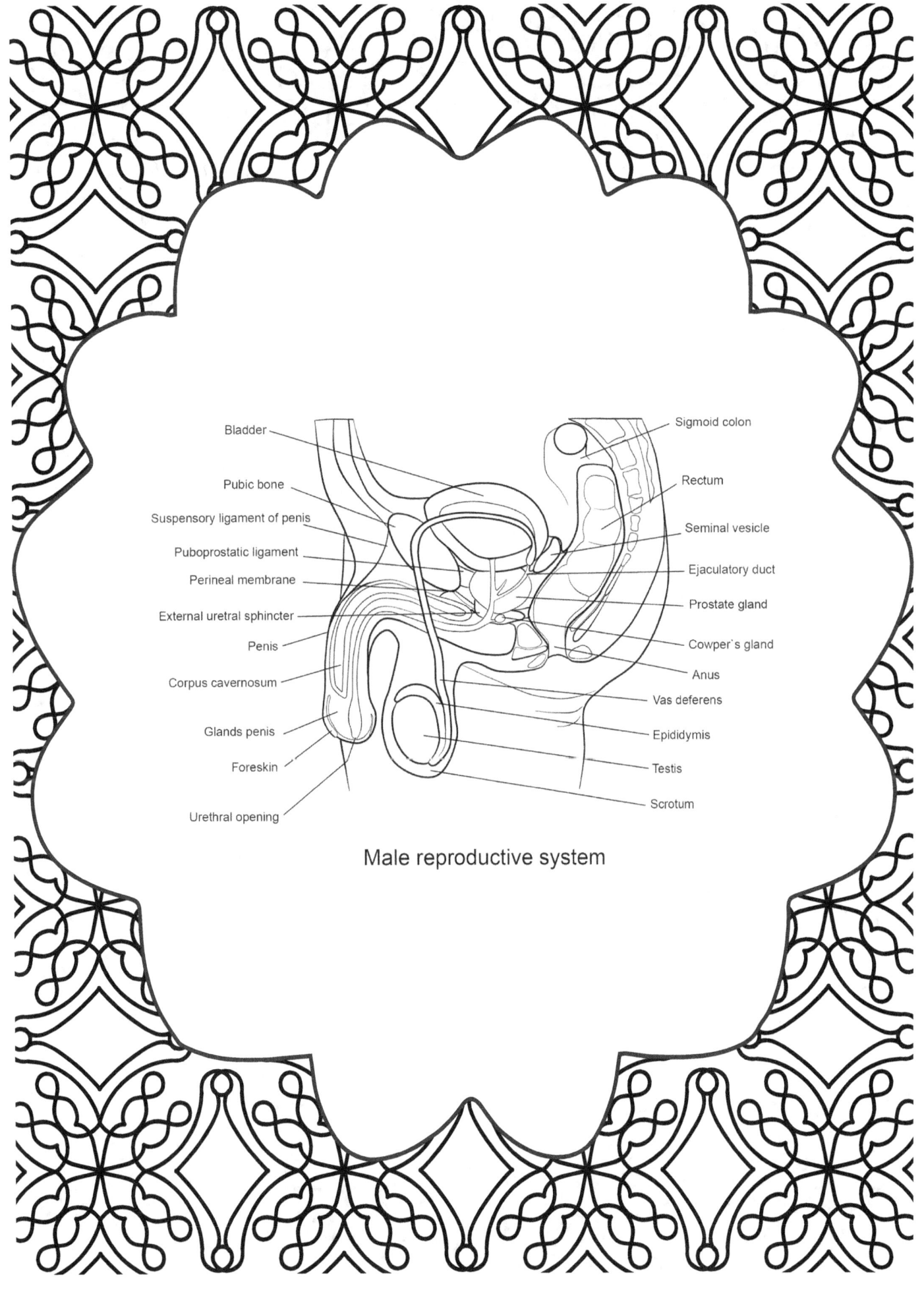

Male reproductive system

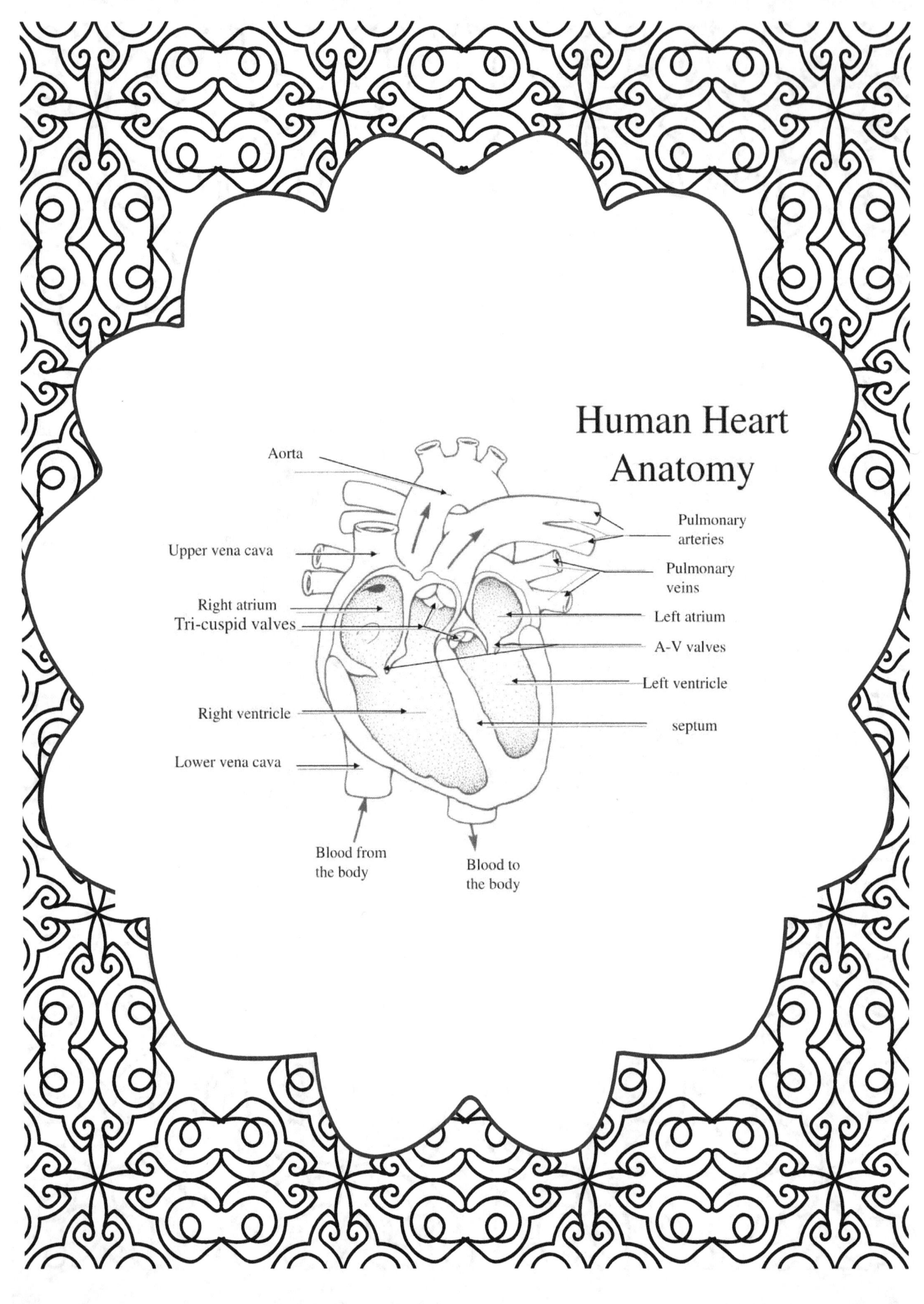

Human Heart Anatomy

Aorta

Pulmonary arteries

Upper vena cava

Pulmonary veins

Right atrium

Tri-cuspid valves

Left atrium

A-V valves

Left ventricle

Right ventricle

septum

Lower vena cava

Blood from the body

Blood to the body

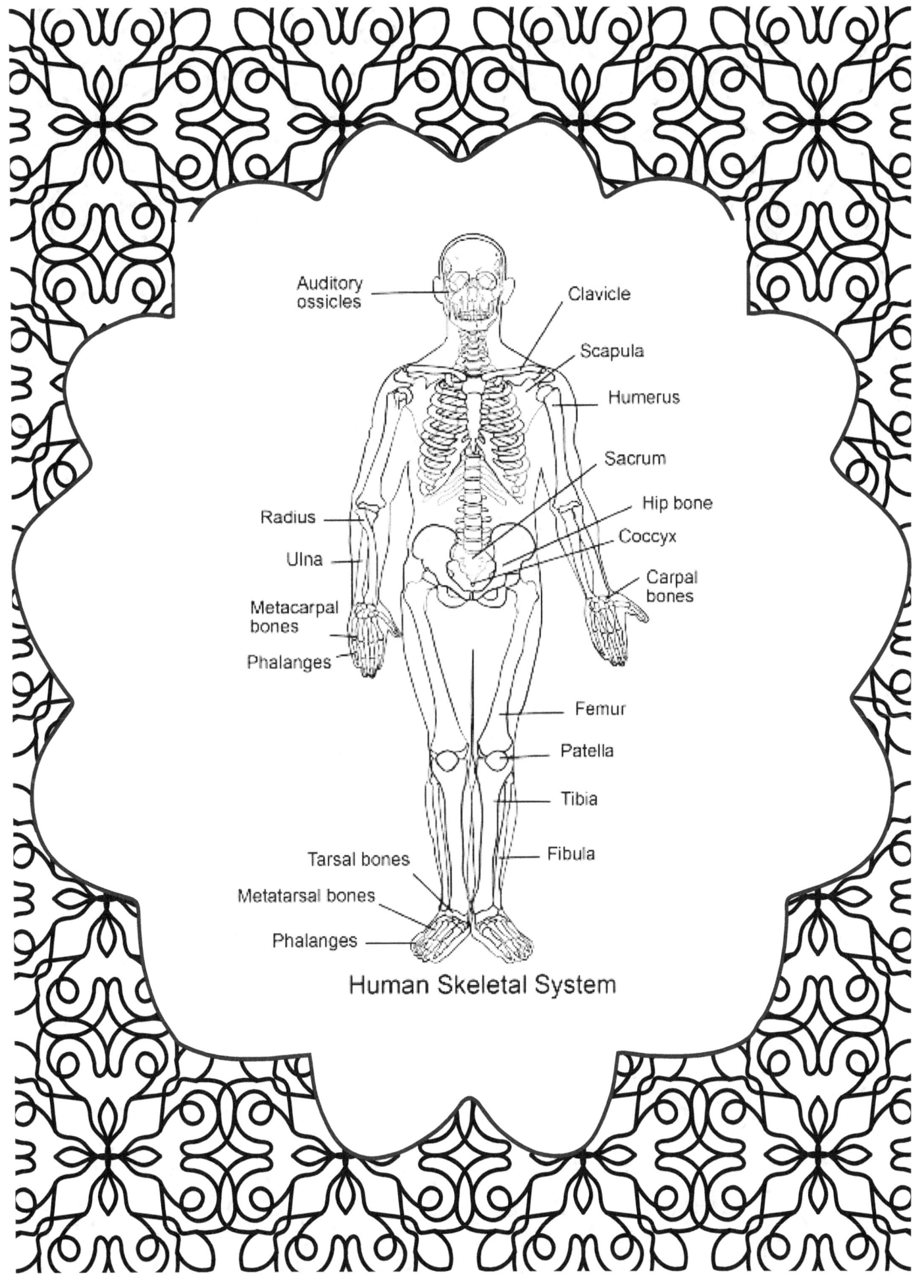

Auditory ossicles

Clavicle

Scapula

Humerus

Sacrum

Hip bone

Coccyx

Carpal bones

Radius

Ulna

Metacarpal bones

Phalanges

Femur

Patella

Tibia

Fibula

Tarsal bones

Metatarsal bones

Phalanges

Human Skeletal System

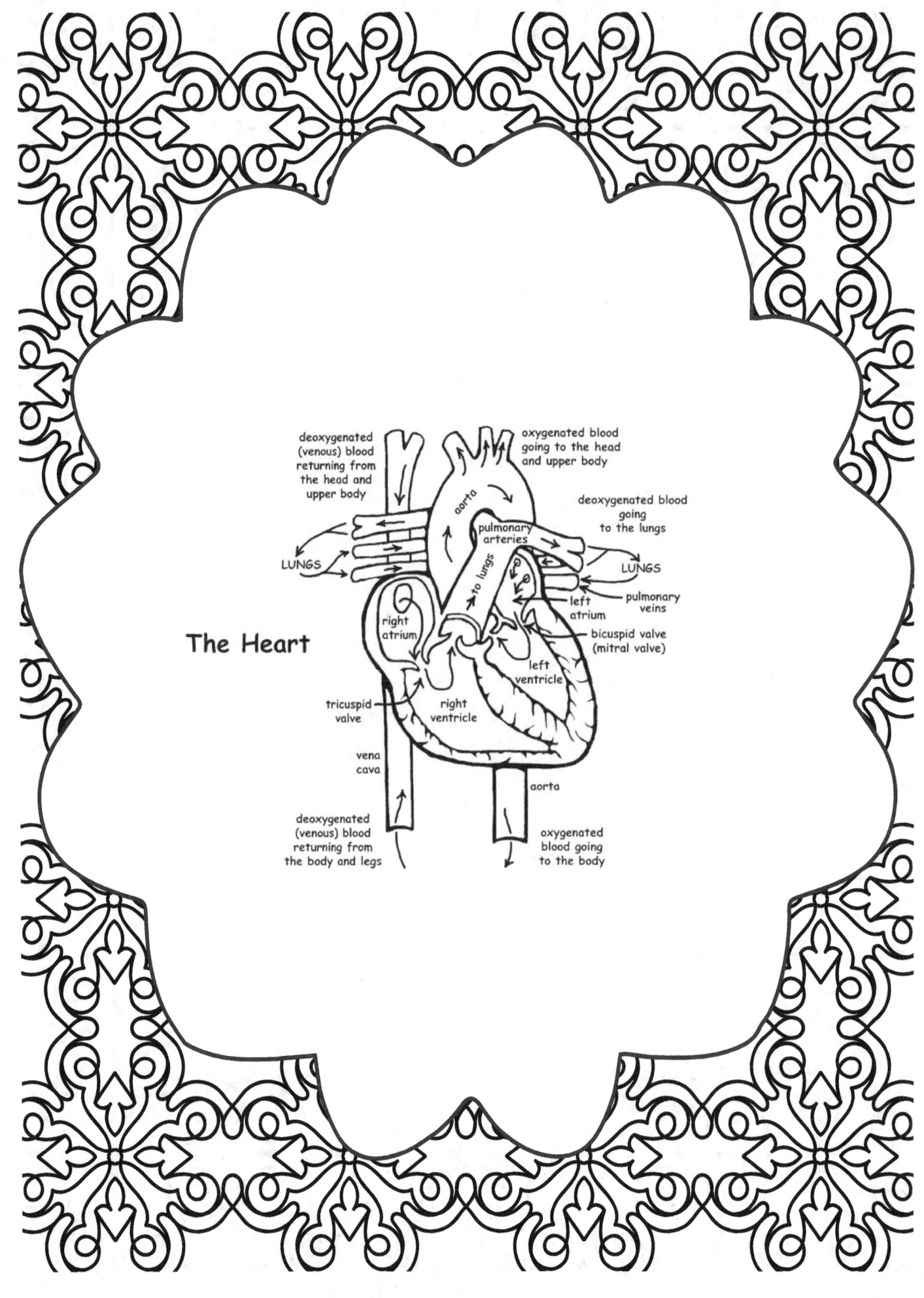

The Heart

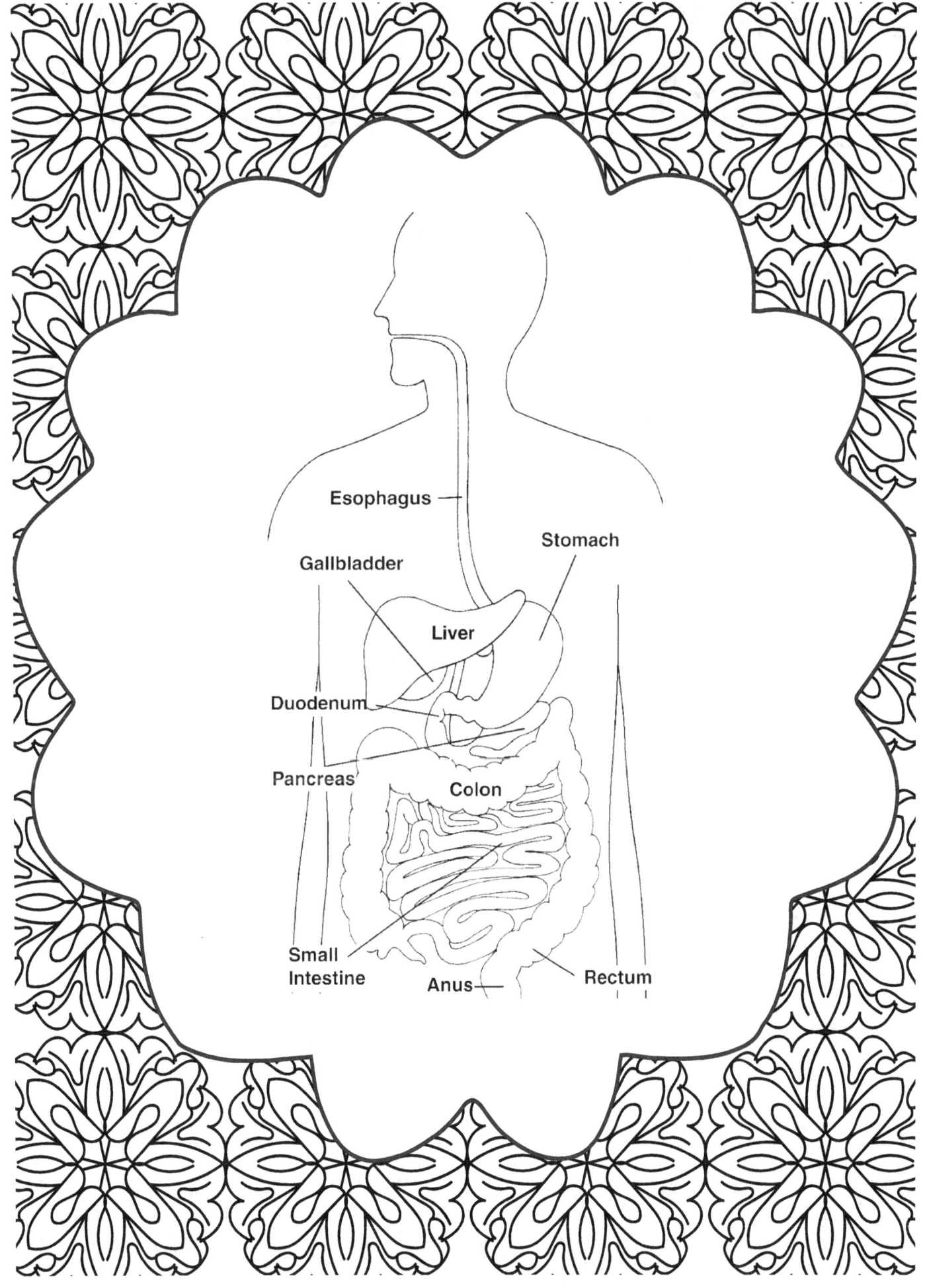

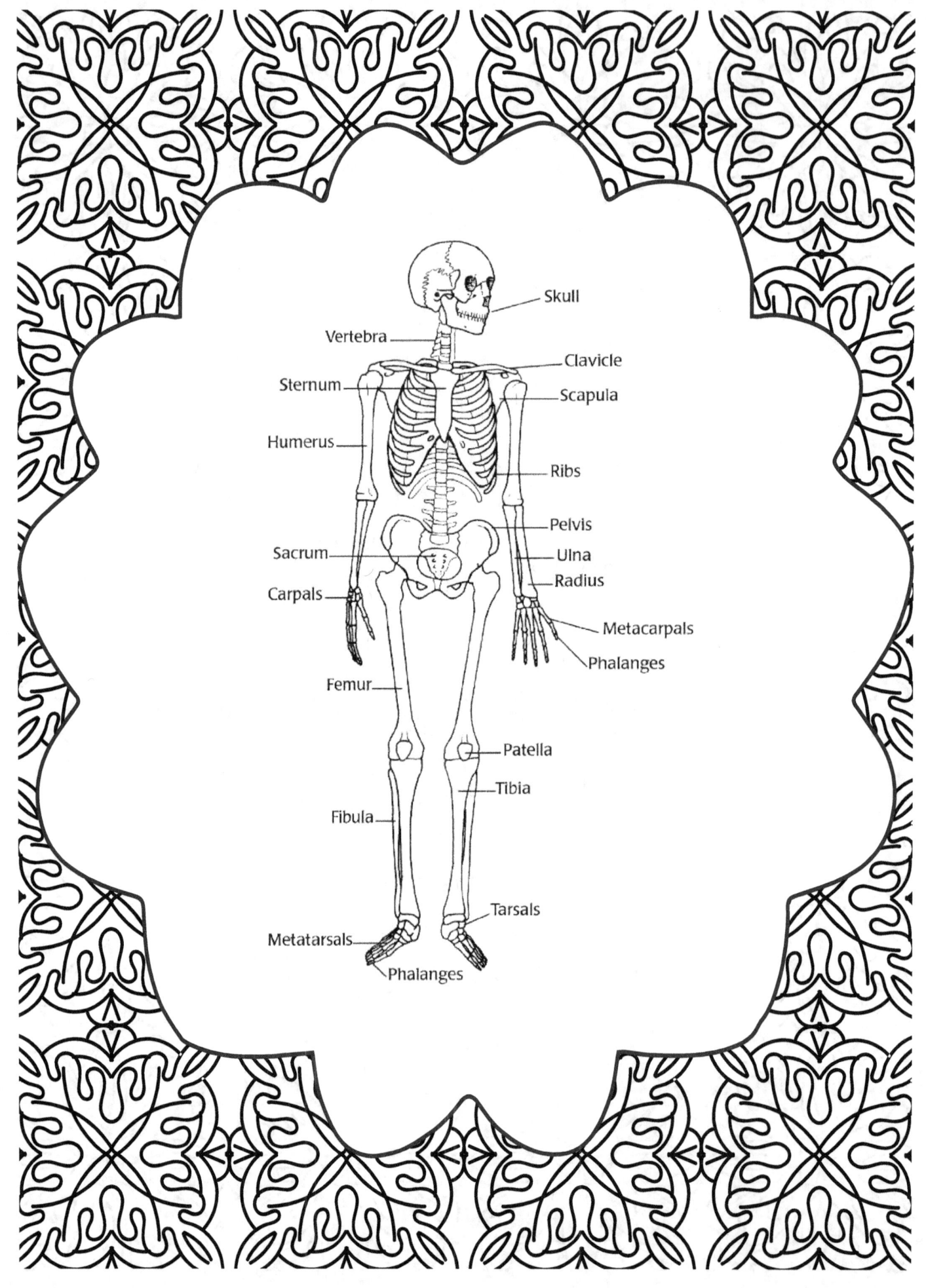

parts of an ear

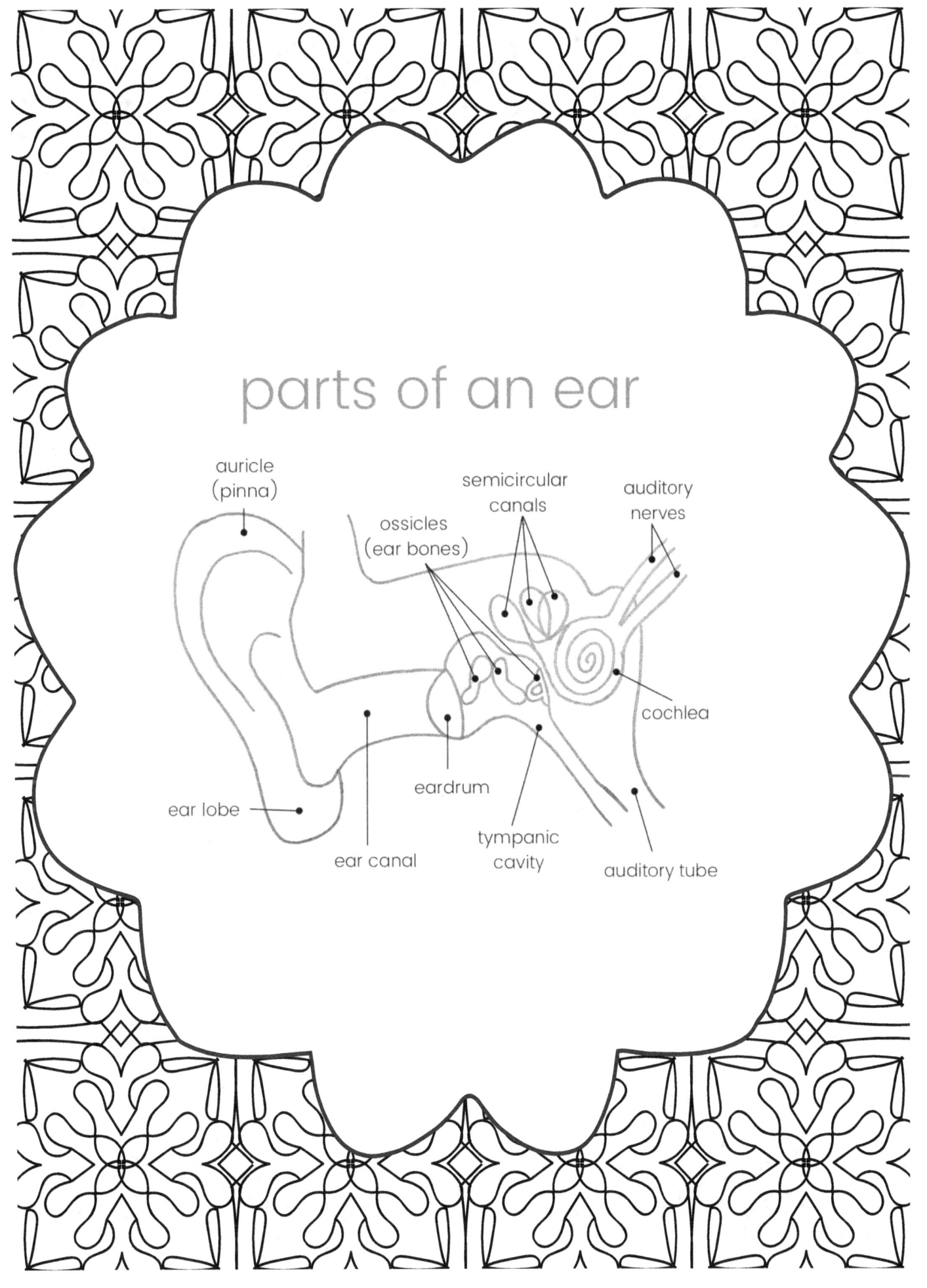

auricle
(pinna)

ossicles
(ear bones)

semicircular
canals

auditory
nerves

cochlea

ear lobe

ear canal

eardrum

tympanic
cavity

auditory tube

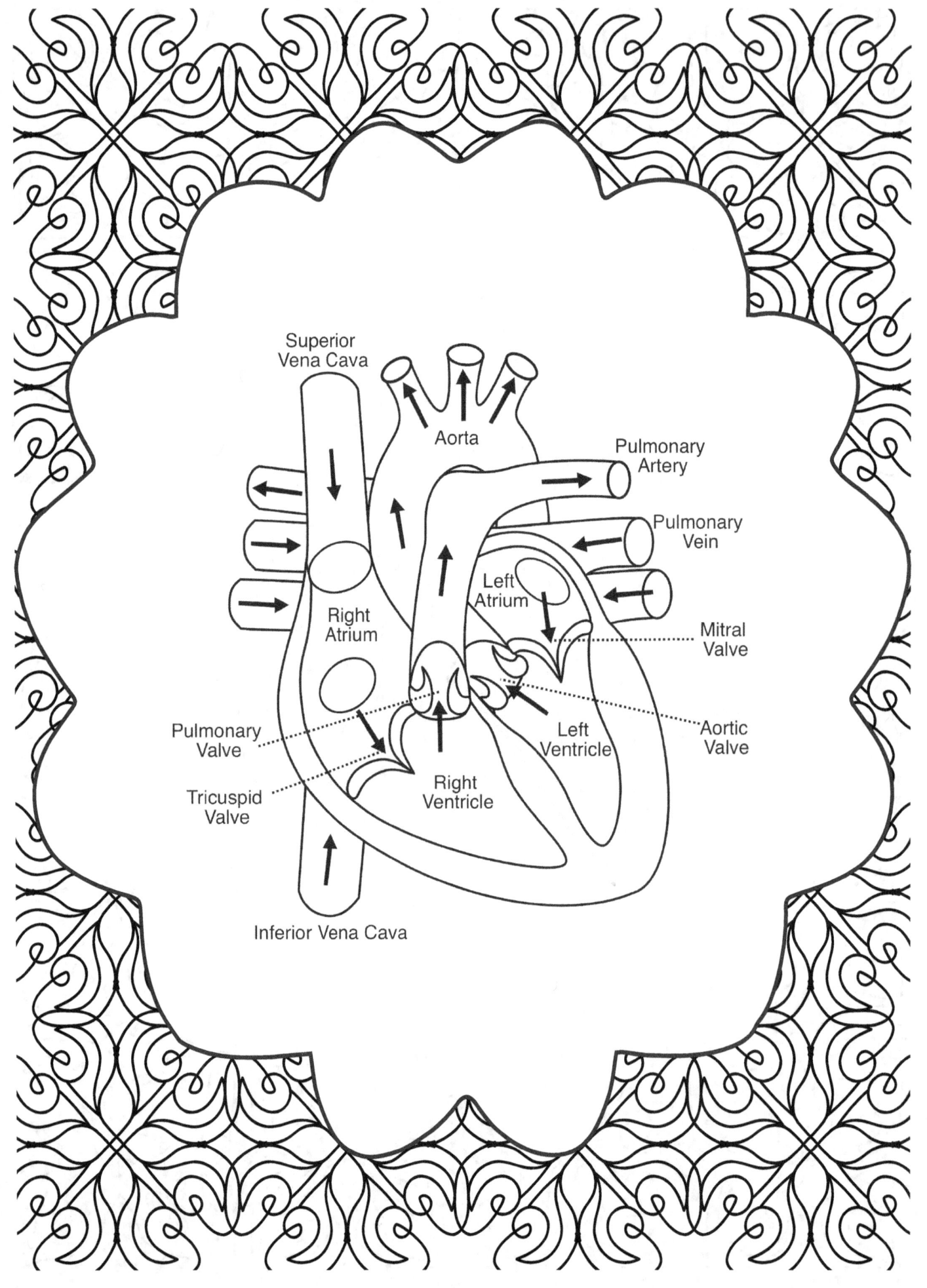

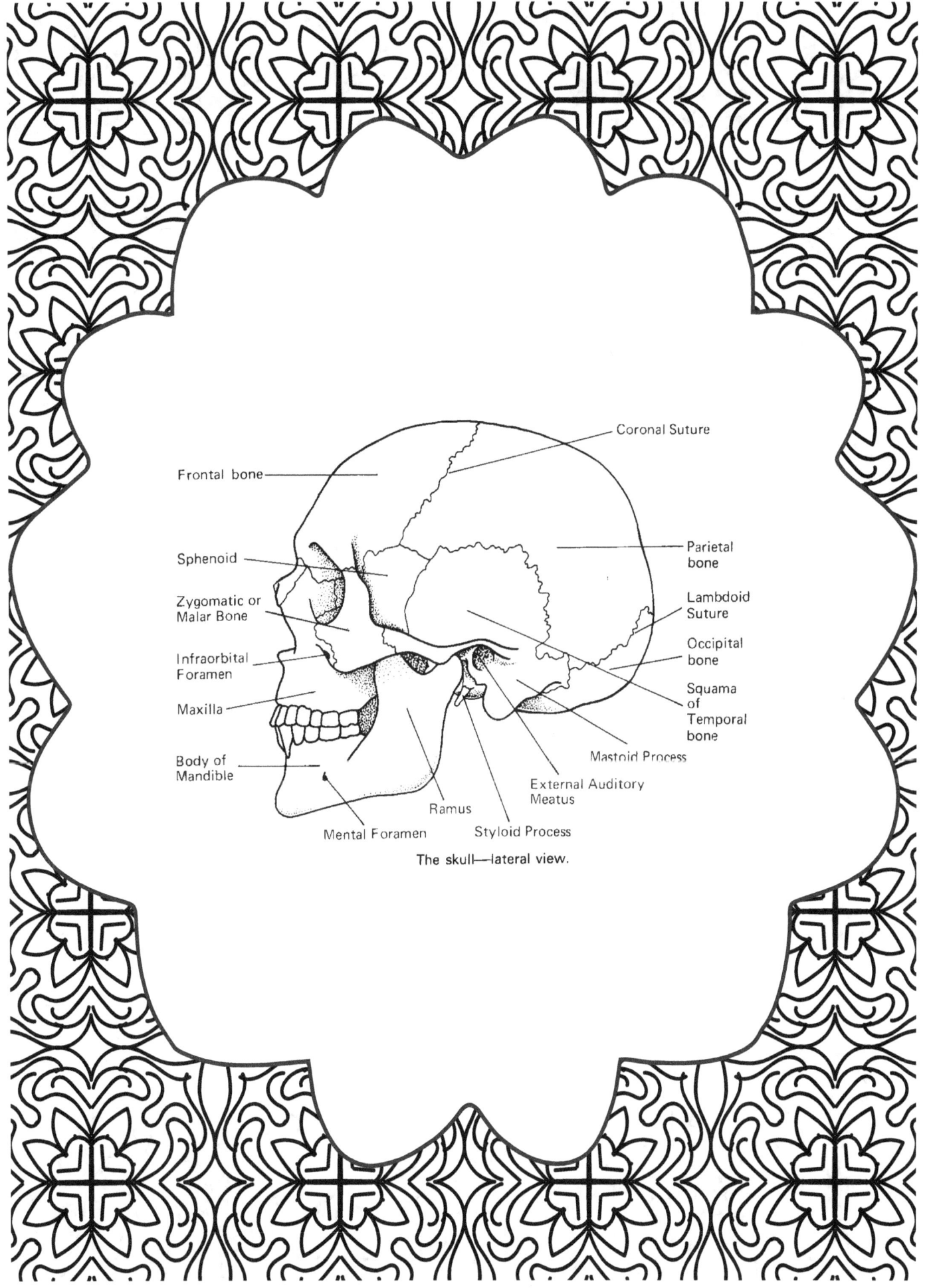

Coronal Suture

Frontal bone

Parietal bone

Sphenoid

Zygomatic or Malar Bone

Lambdoid Suture

Occipital bone

Infraorbital Foramen

Squama of Temporal bone

Maxilla

Body of Mandible

Mastoid Process

External Auditory Meatus

Ramus

Mental Foramen

Styloid Process

The skull—lateral view.

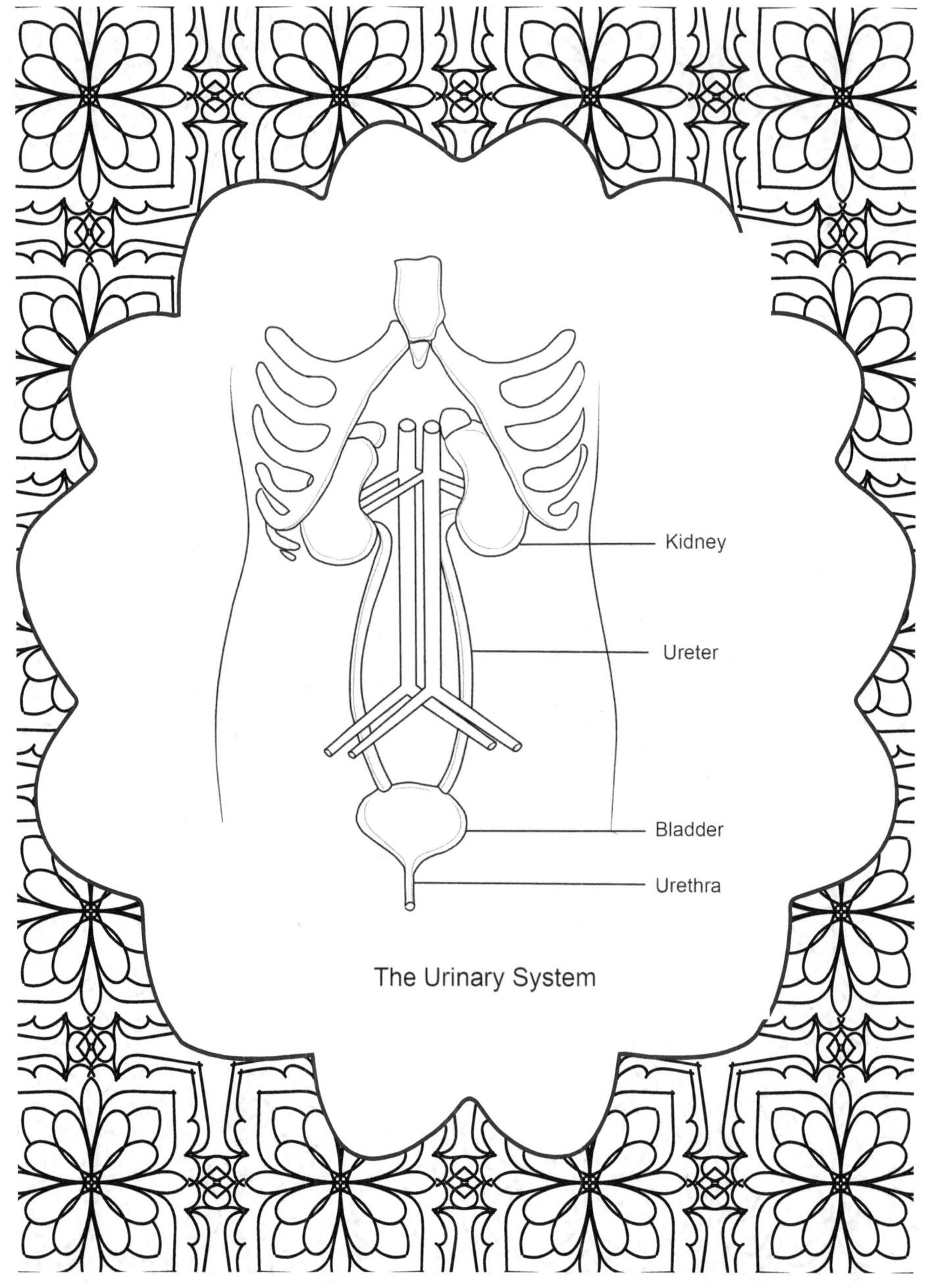

Kidney

Ureter

Bladder

Urethra

The Urinary System

Anatomy of the Eye

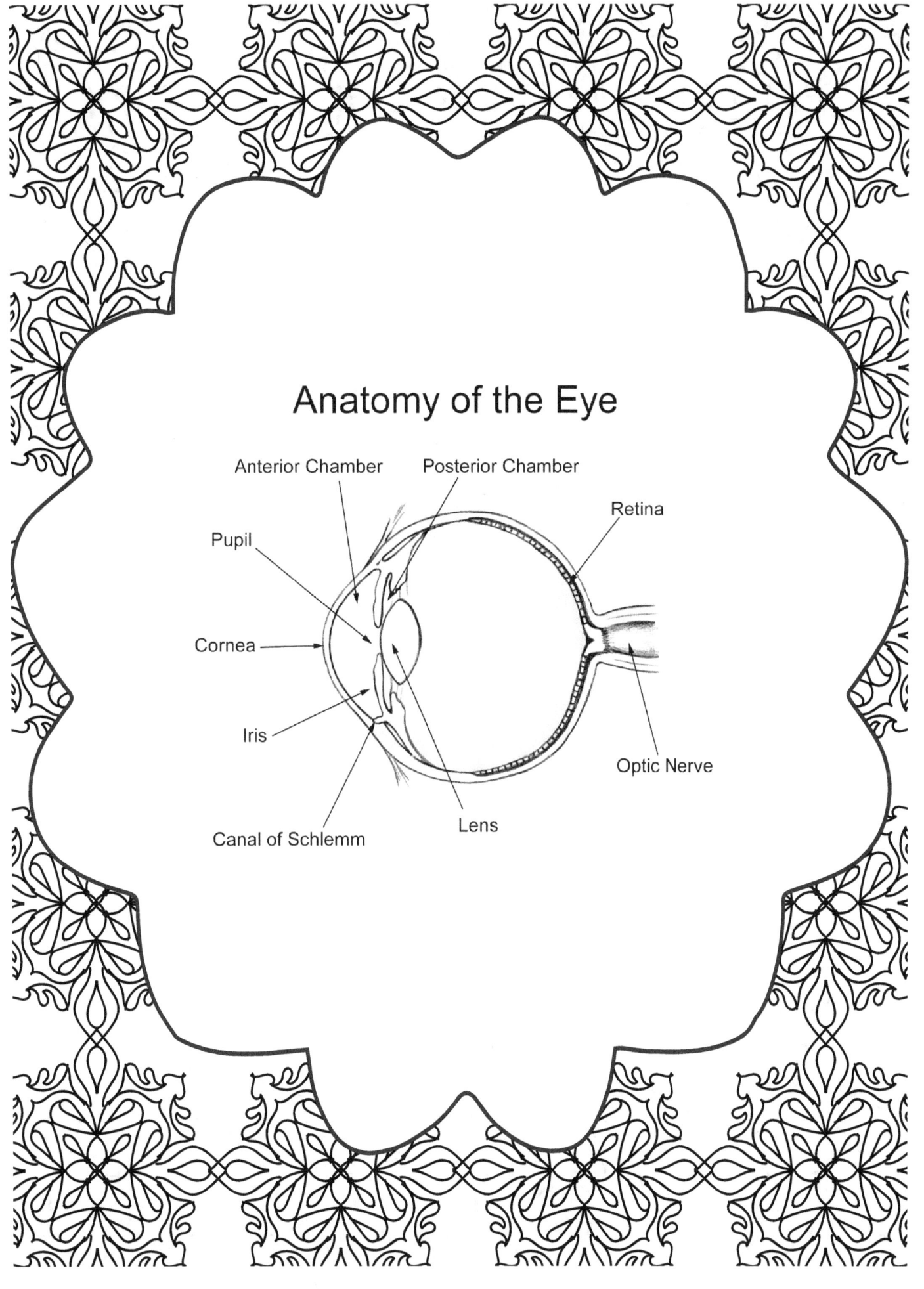

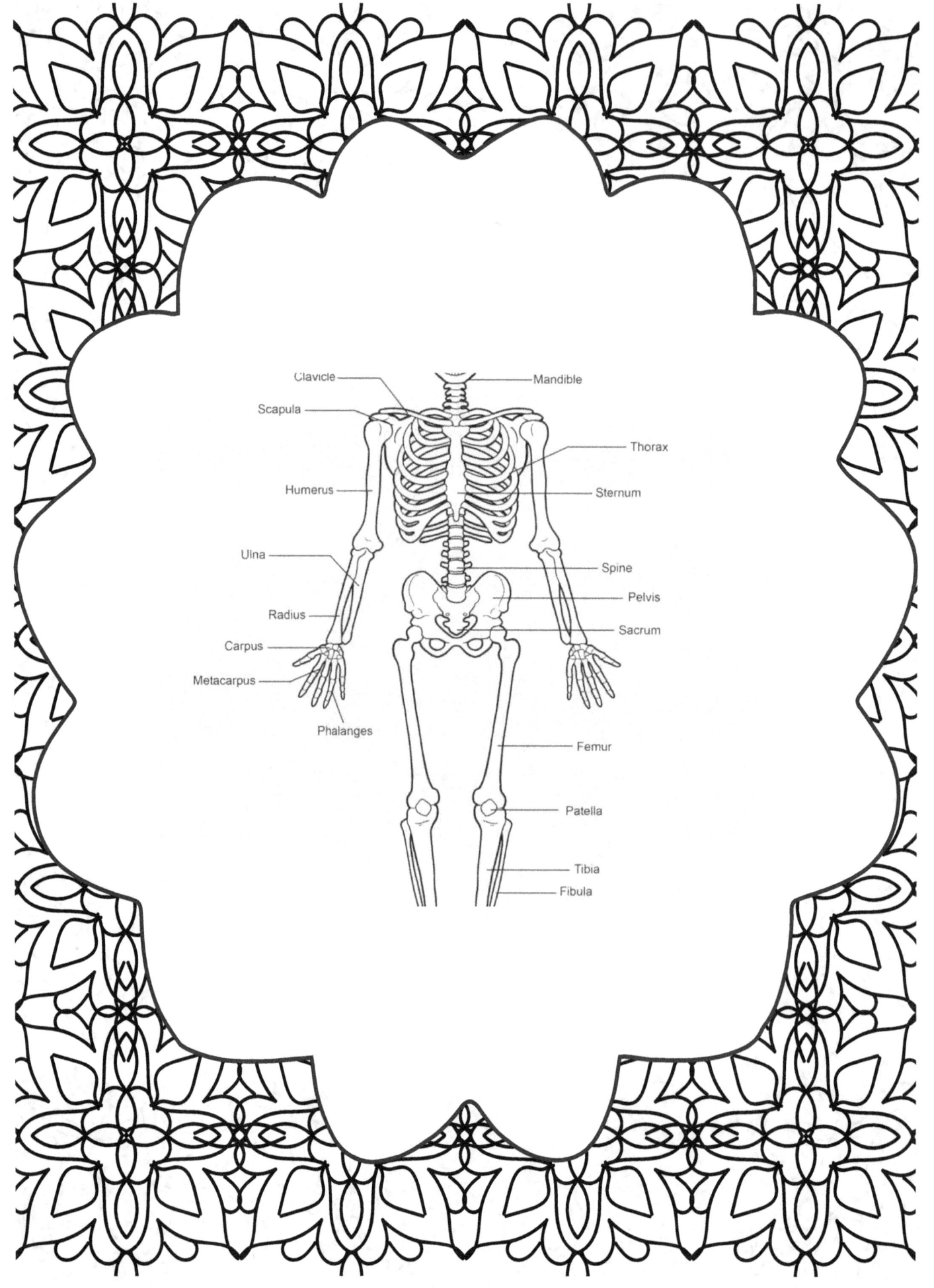

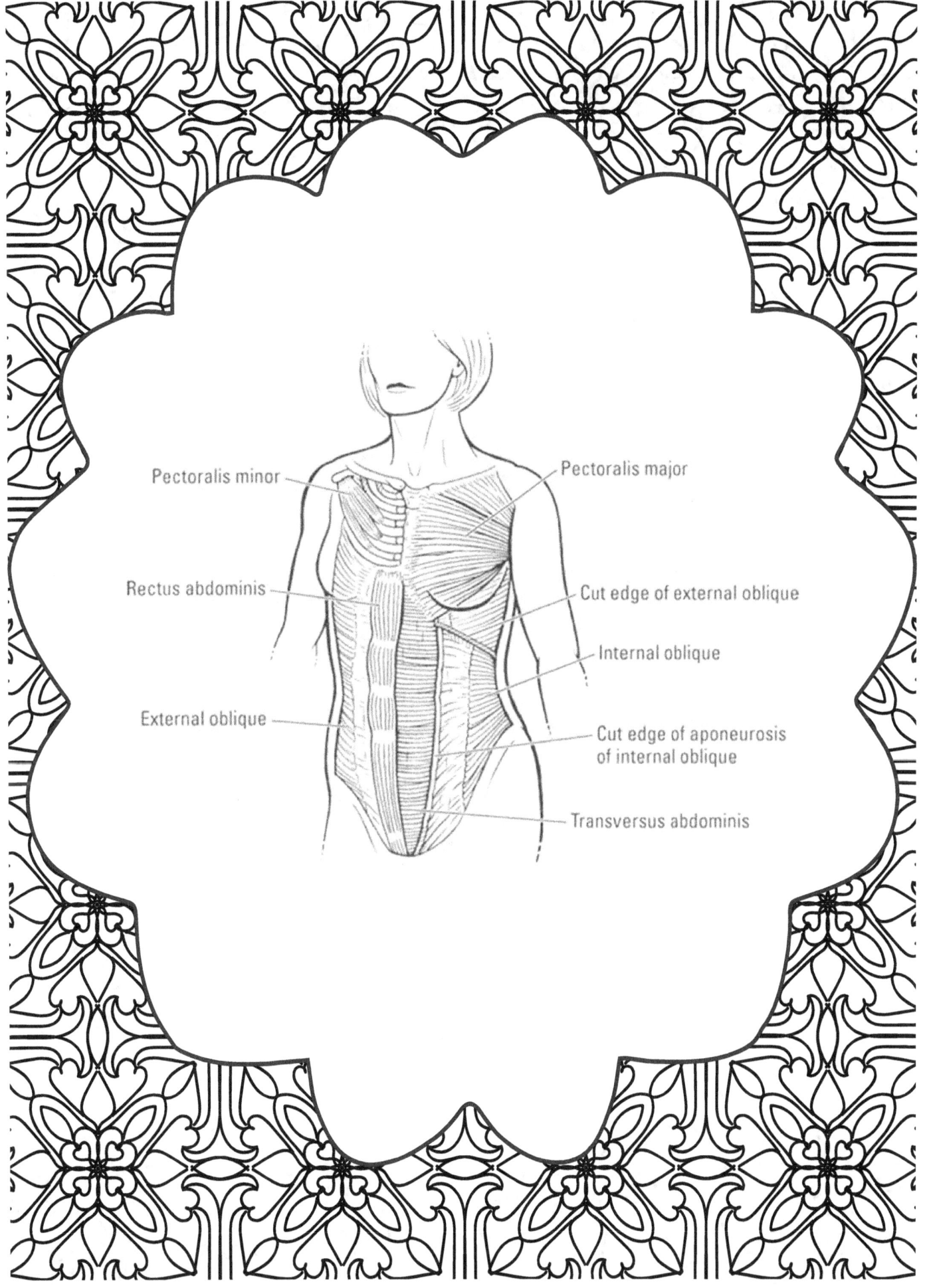

Pectoralis minor

Pectoralis major

Rectus abdominis

Cut edge of external oblique

Internal oblique

External oblique

Cut edge of aponeurosis
of internal oblique

Transversus abdominis

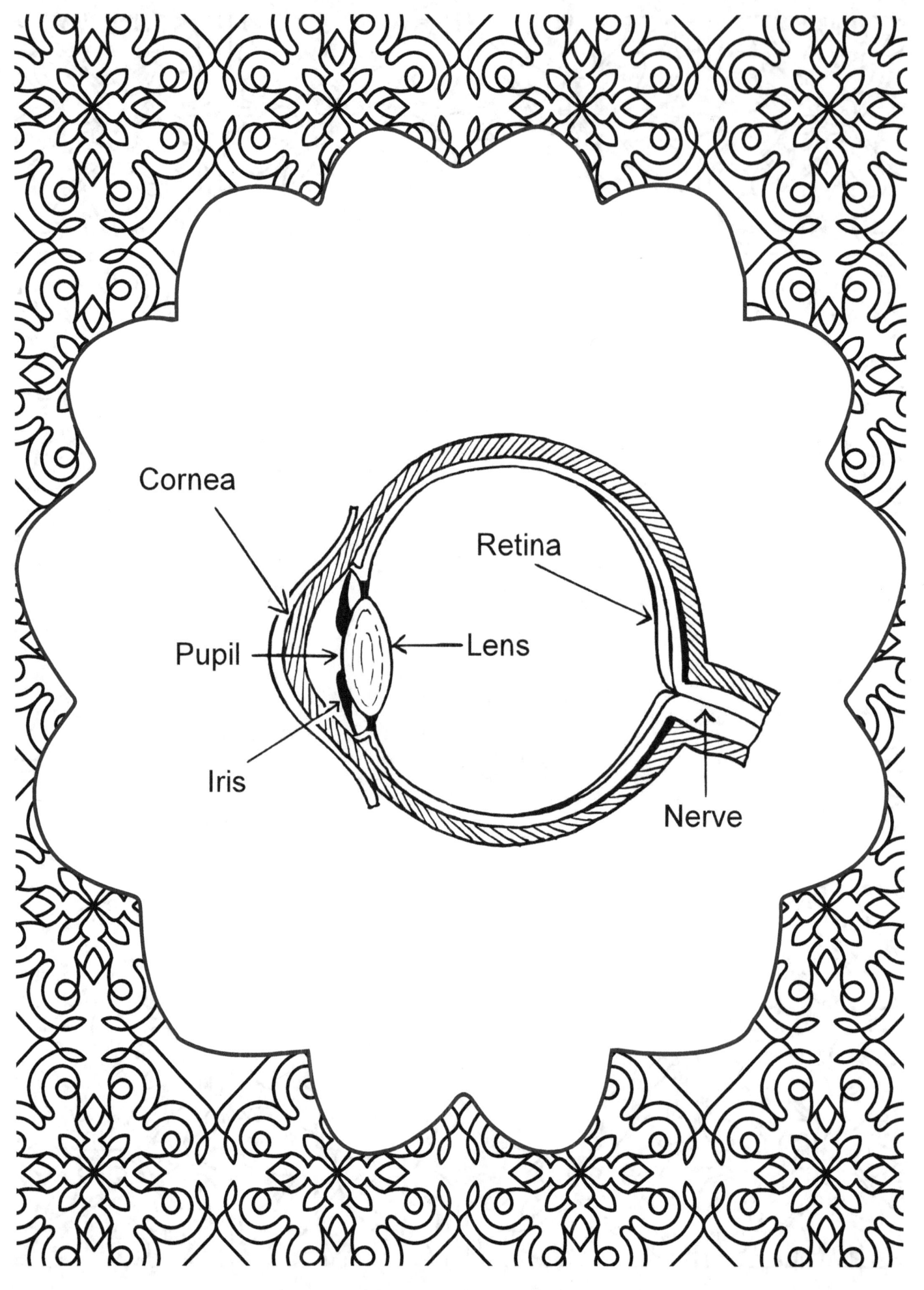

Cornea

Retina

Pupil

Lens

Iris

Nerve

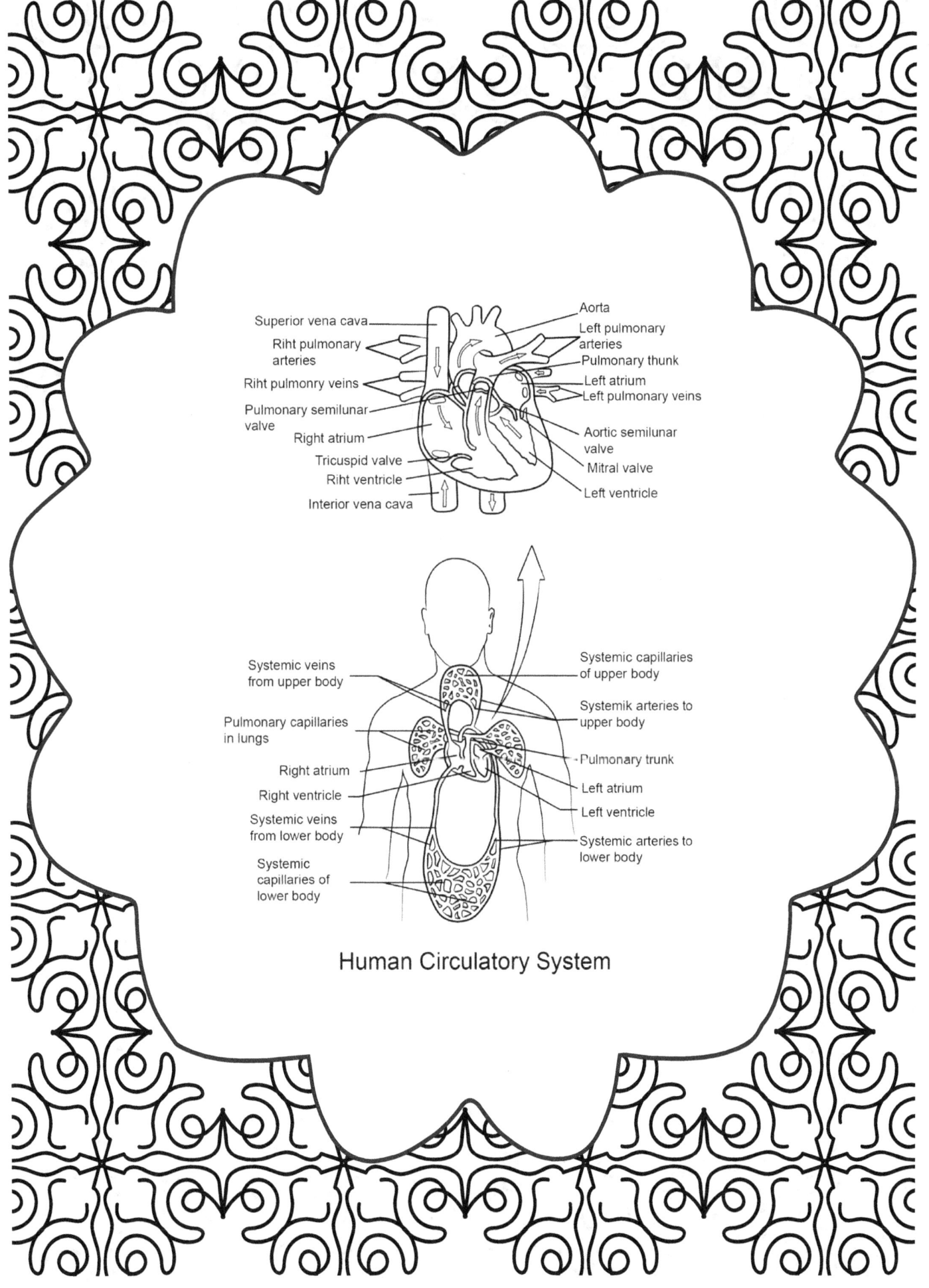

Human Circulatory System

Internal structure of the brain

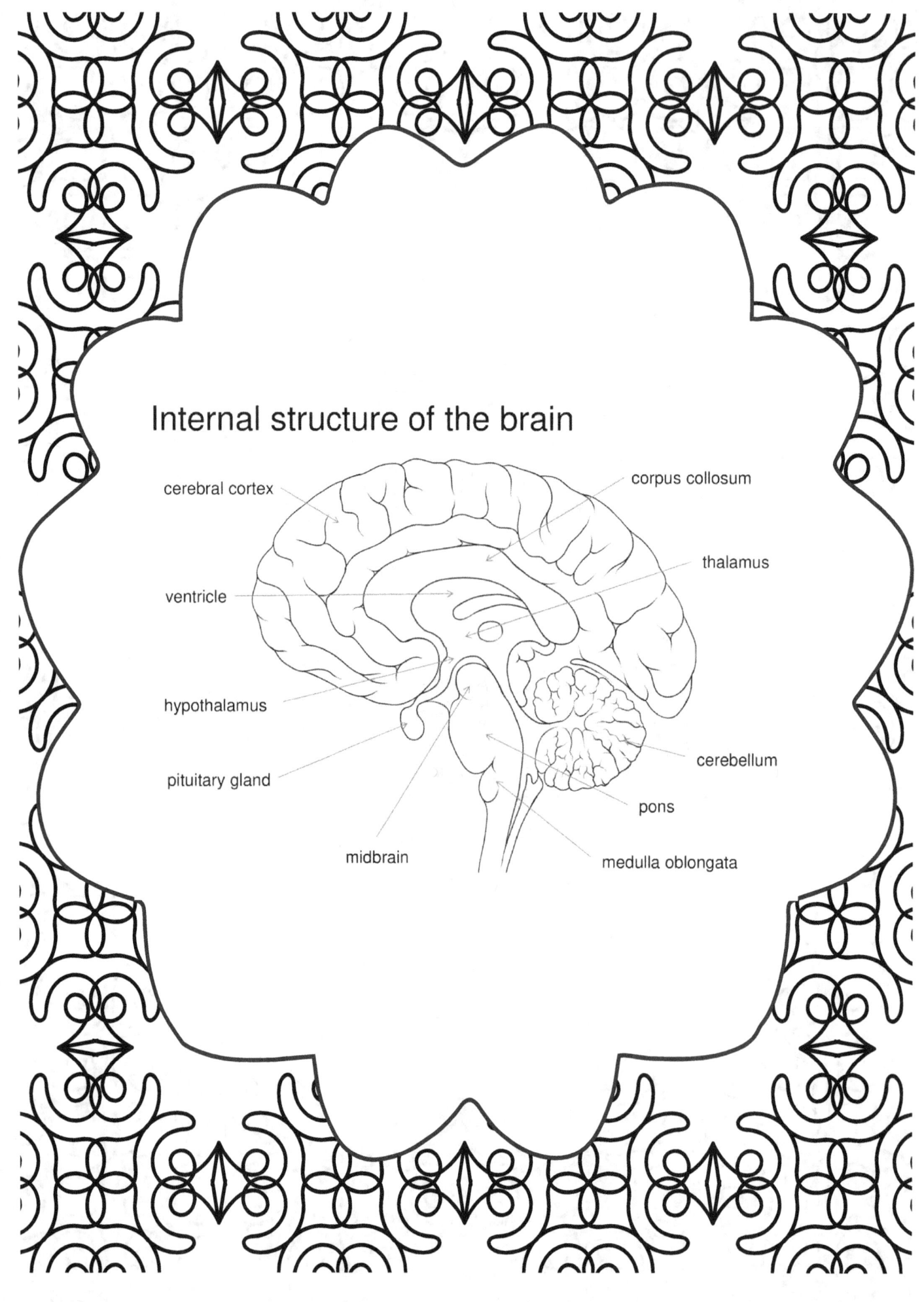

cerebral cortex

corpus collosum

thalamus

ventricle

hypothalamus

pituitary gland

cerebellum

pons

midbrain

medulla oblongata

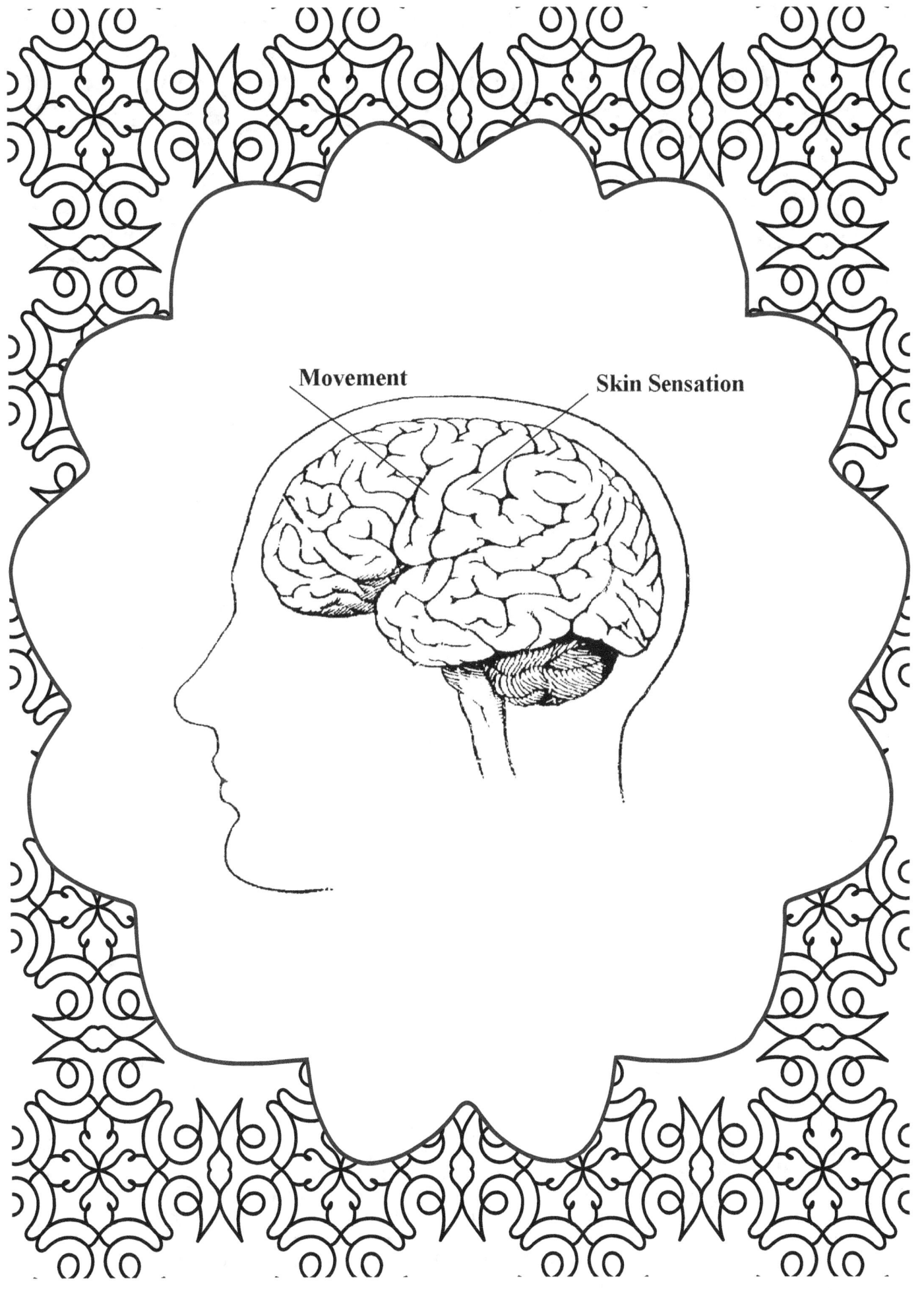

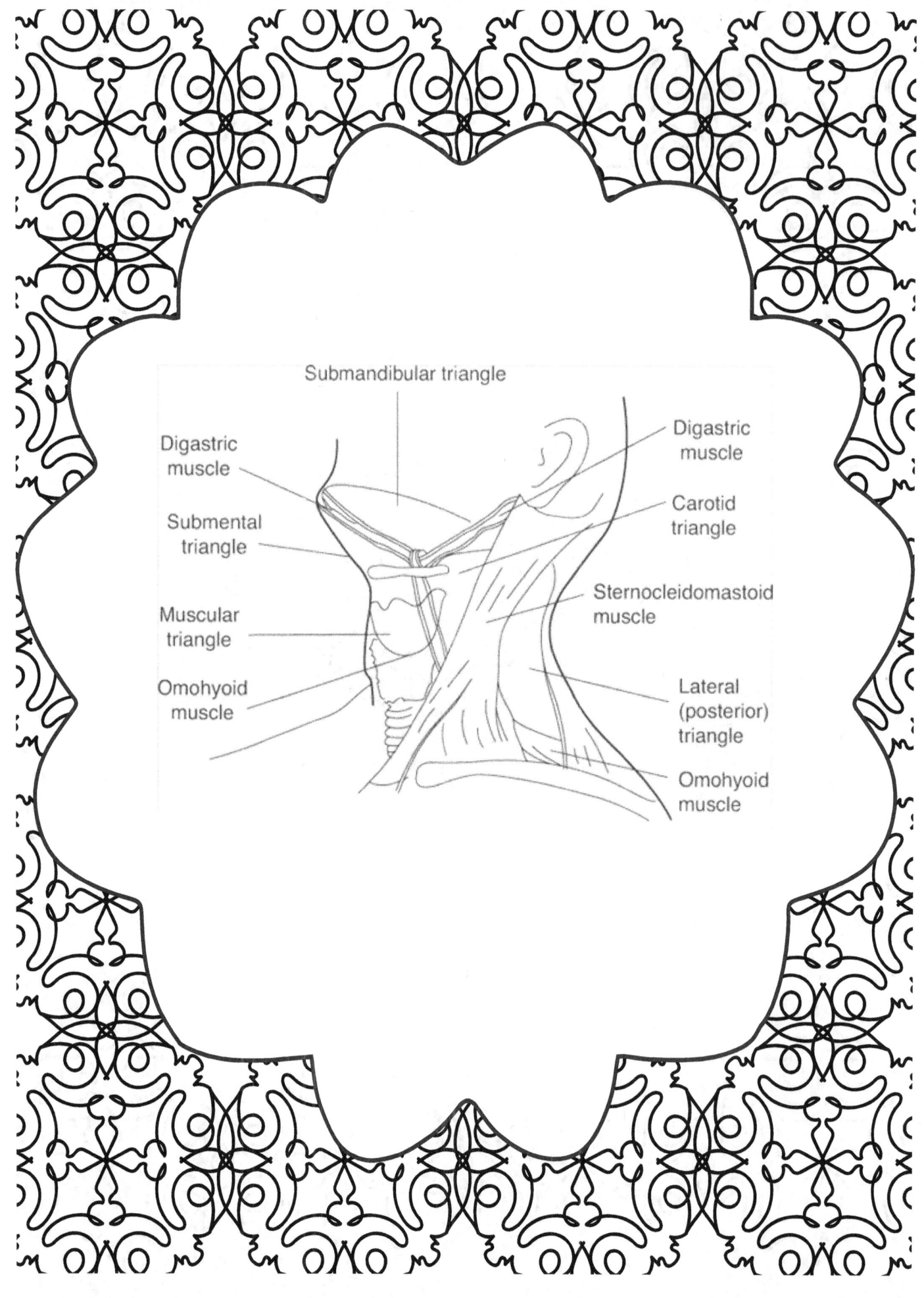

Submandibular triangle

Digastric muscle

Submental triangle

Muscular triangle

Omohyoid muscle

Digastric muscle

Carotid triangle

Sternocleidomastoid muscle

Lateral (posterior) triangle

Omohyoid muscle

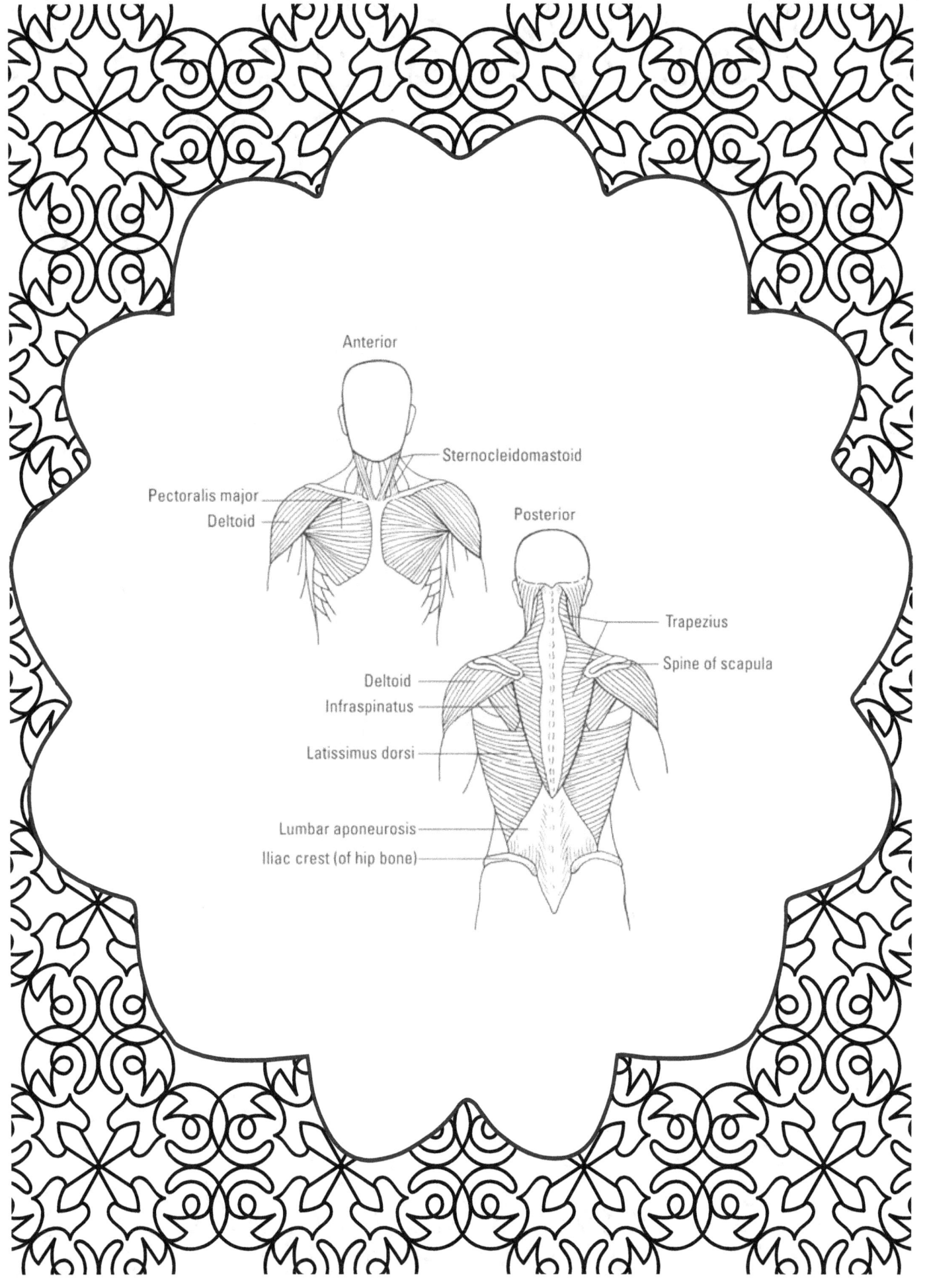

Anterior

Sternocleidomastoid

Pectoralis major

Deltoid

Posterior

Trapezius

Spine of scapula

Deltoid

Infraspinatus

Latissimus dorsi

Lumbar aponeurosis

Iliac crest (of hip bone)

Color the Digestive Tract

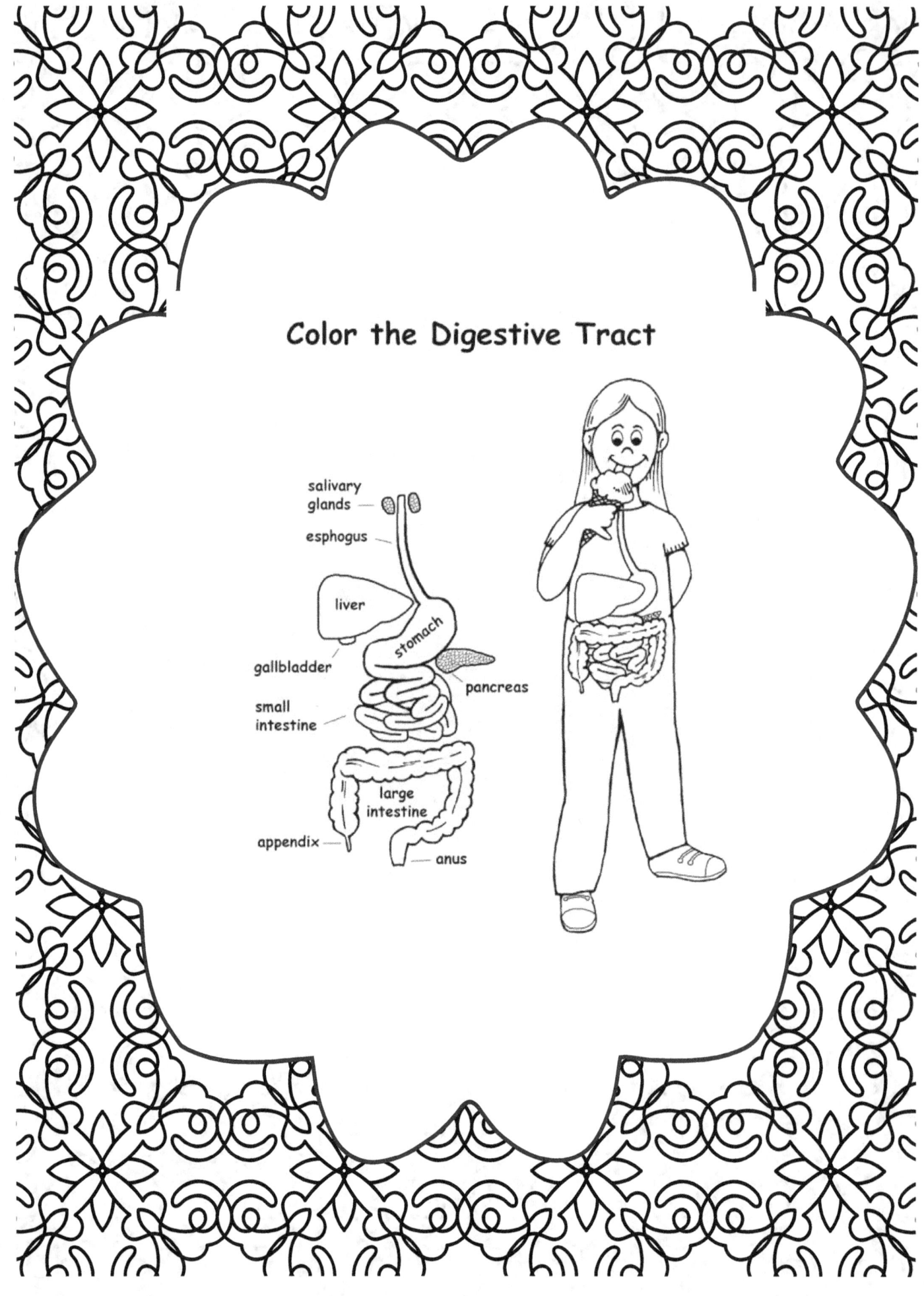

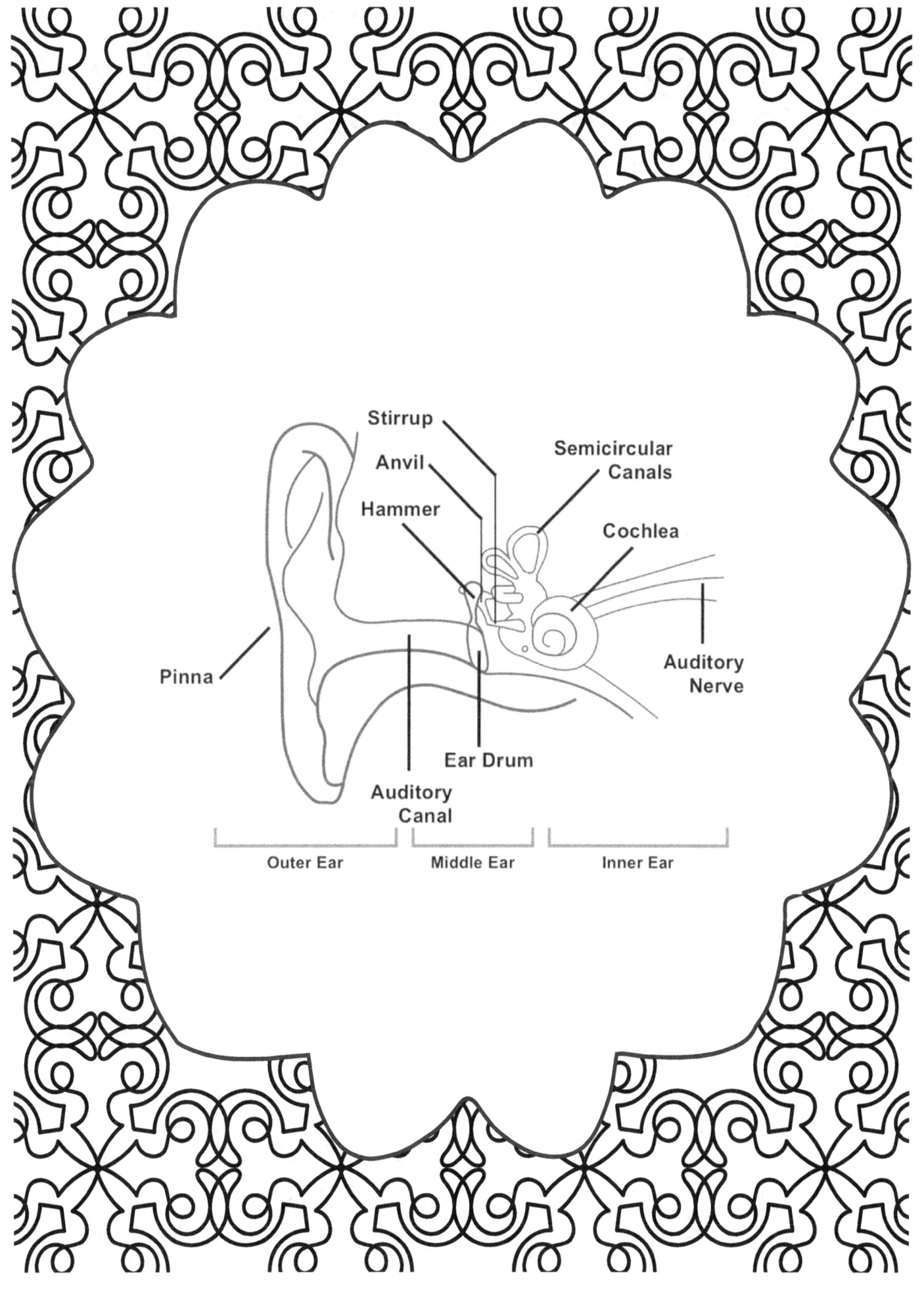

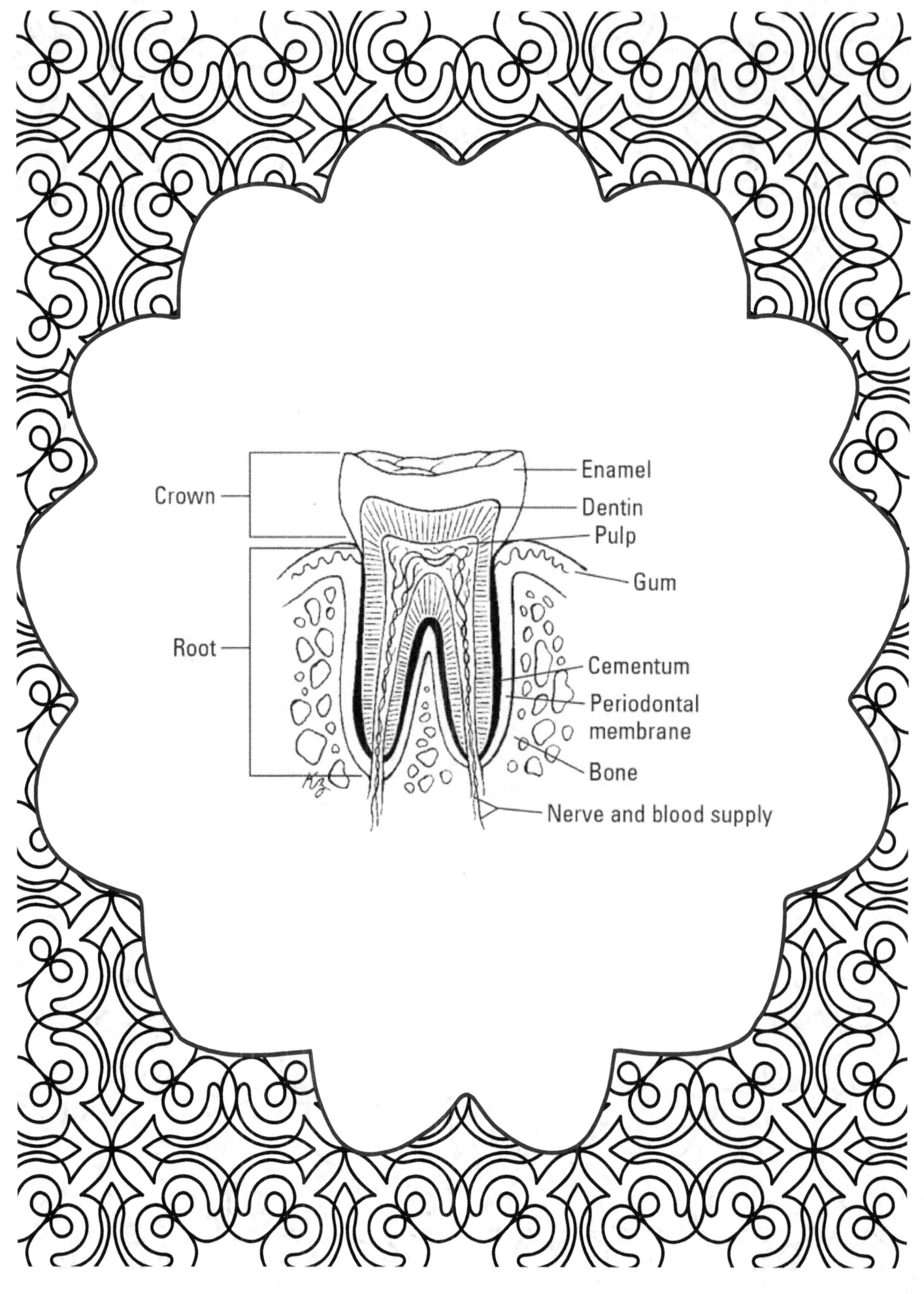

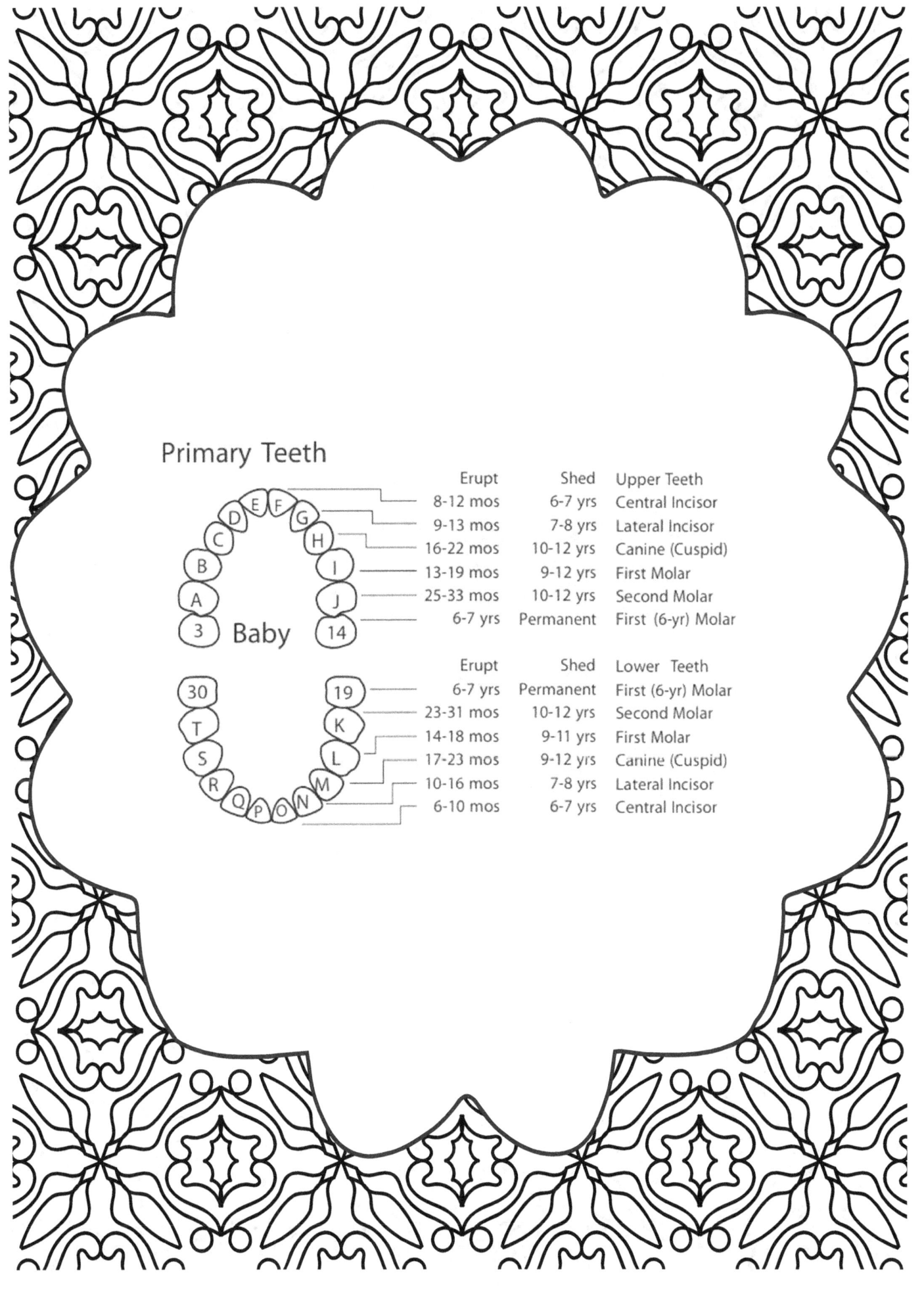

Primary Teeth

	Erupt	Shed	Upper Teeth
	8-12 mos	6-7 yrs	Central Incisor
	9-13 mos	7-8 yrs	Lateral Incisor
	16-22 mos	10-12 yrs	Canine (Cuspid)
	13-19 mos	9-12 yrs	First Molar
	25-33 mos	10-12 yrs	Second Molar
	6-7 yrs	Permanent	First (6-yr) Molar

	Erupt	Shed	Lower Teeth
	6-7 yrs	Permanent	First (6-yr) Molar
	23-31 mos	10-12 yrs	Second Molar
	14-18 mos	9-11 yrs	First Molar
	17-23 mos	9-12 yrs	Canine (Cuspid)
	10-16 mos	7-8 yrs	Lateral Incisor
	6-10 mos	6-7 yrs	Central Incisor

Baby

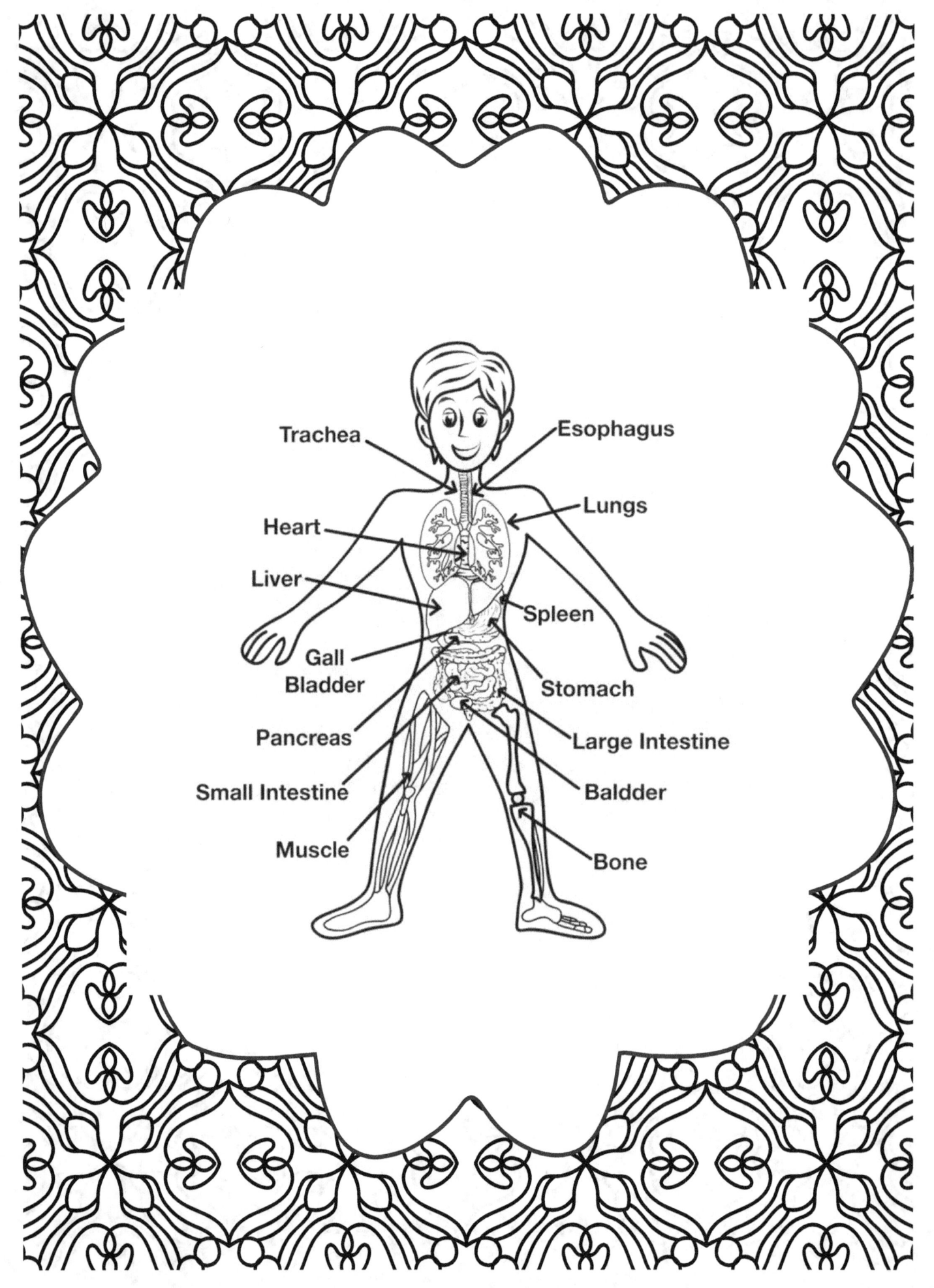

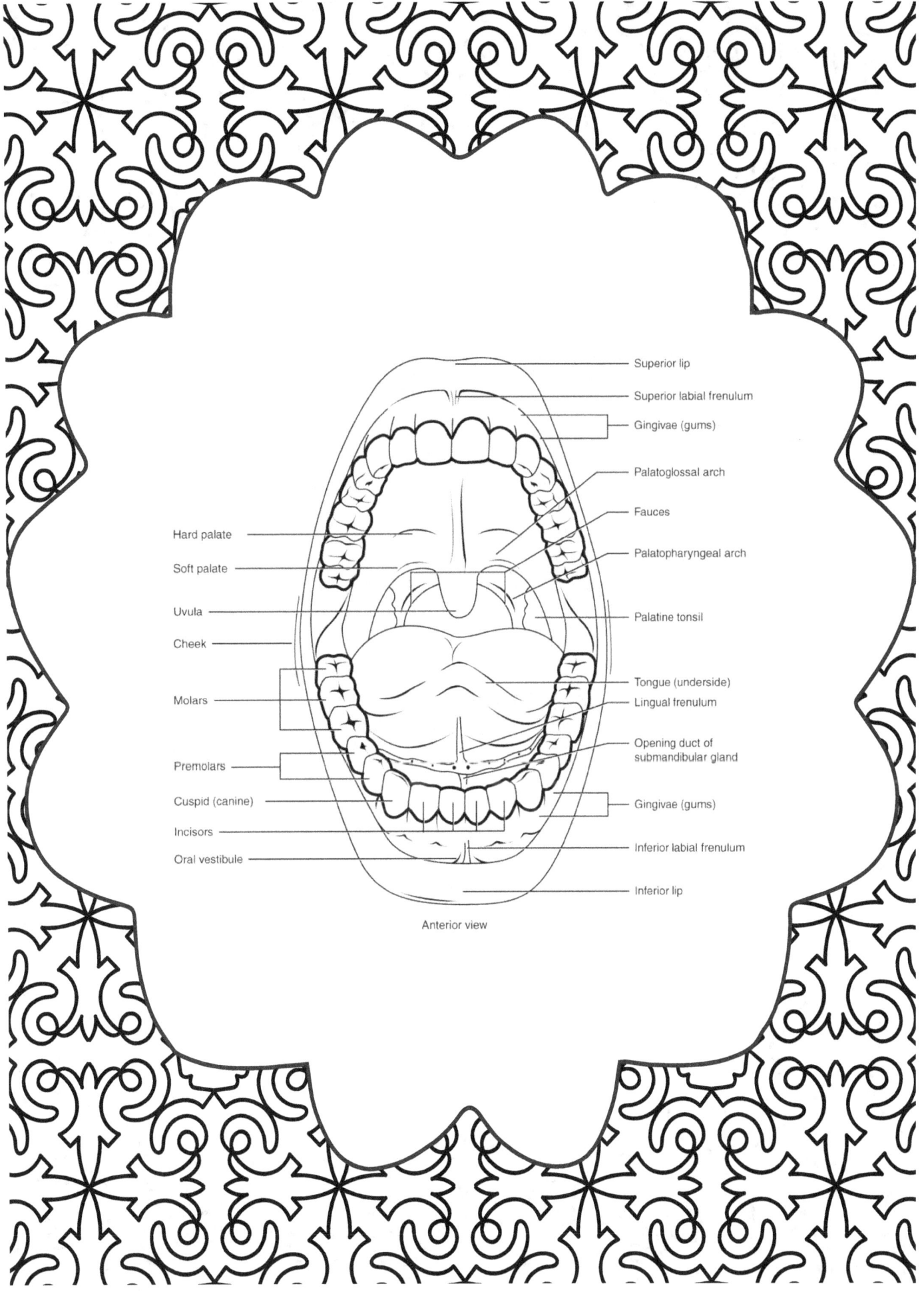

Superior lip

Superior labial frenulum

Gingivae (gums)

Palatoglossal arch

Fauces

Palatopharyngeal arch

Hard palate

Soft palate

Palatine tonsil

Uvula

Cheek

Tongue (underside)

Lingual frenulum

Molars

Opening duct of submandibular gland

Premolars

Cuspid (canine)

Gingivae (gums)

Incisors

Inferior labial frenulum

Oral vestibule

Inferior lip

Anterior view

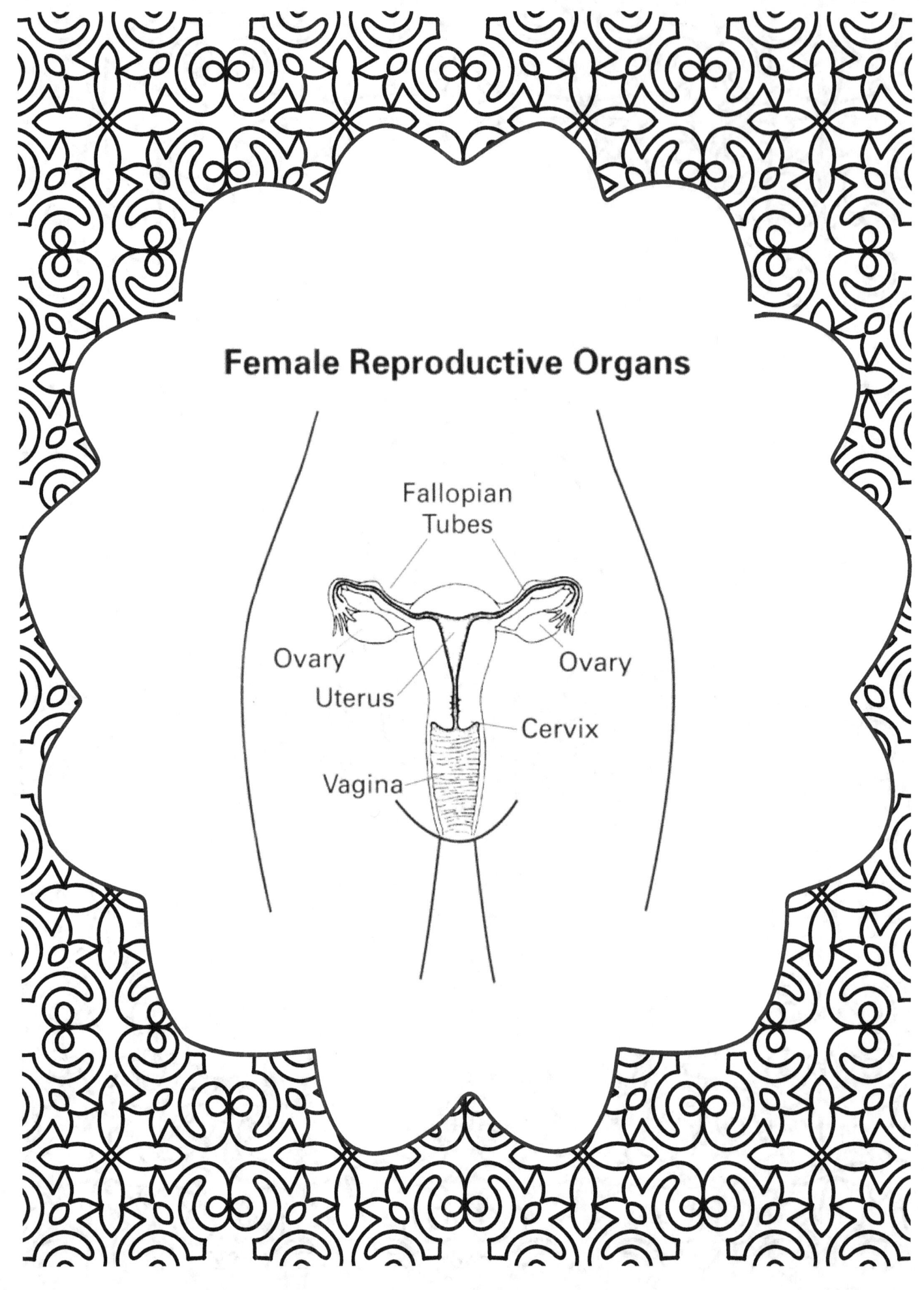

Female Reproductive Organs

Fallopian
Tubes

Ovary

Ovary

Uterus

Cervix

Vagina

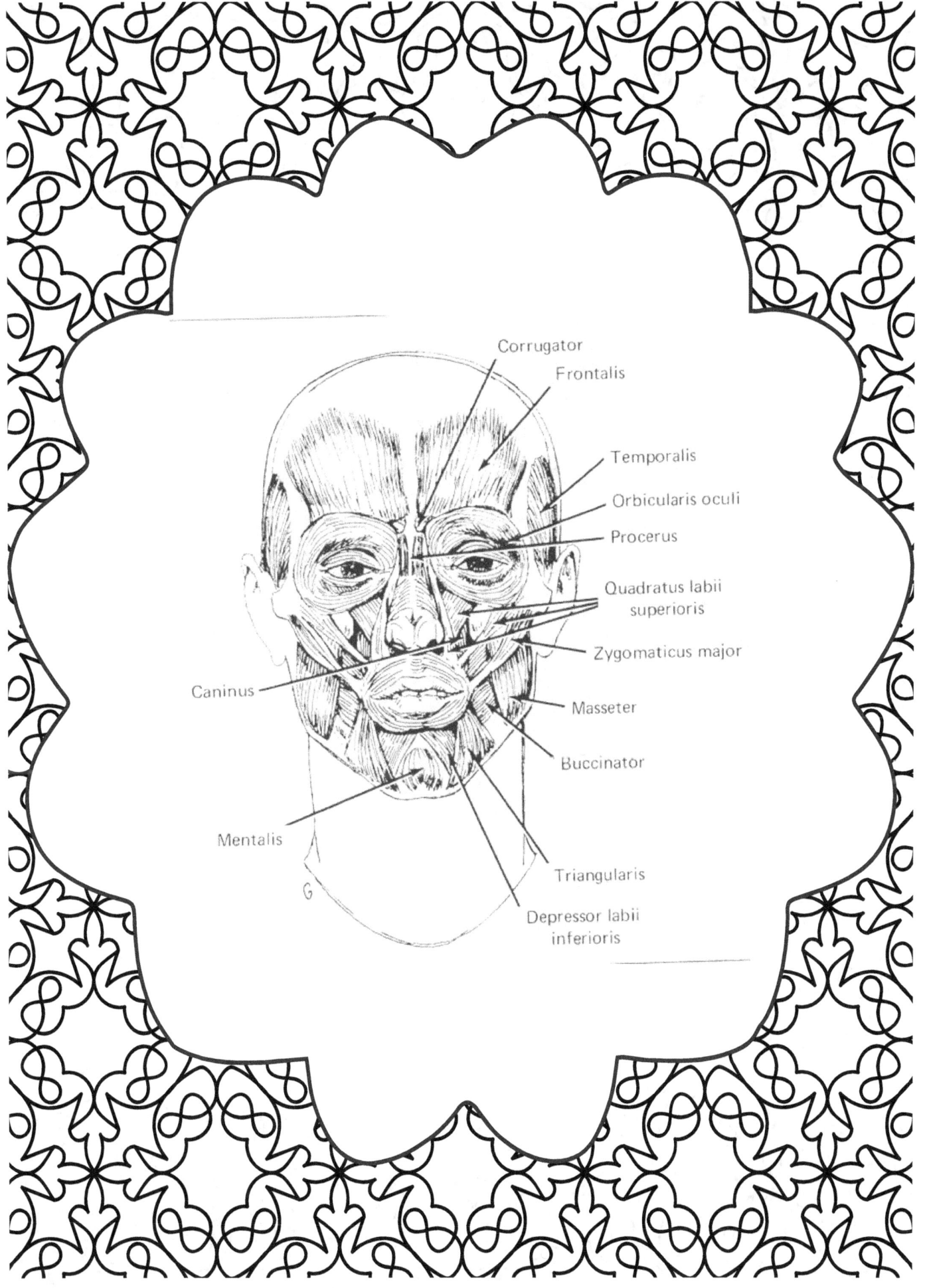

Corrugator

Frontalis

Temporalis

Orbicularis oculi

Procerus

Quadratus labii
superioris

Zygomaticus major

Caninus

Masseter

Buccinator

Mentalis

Triangularis

Depressor labii
inferioris

G

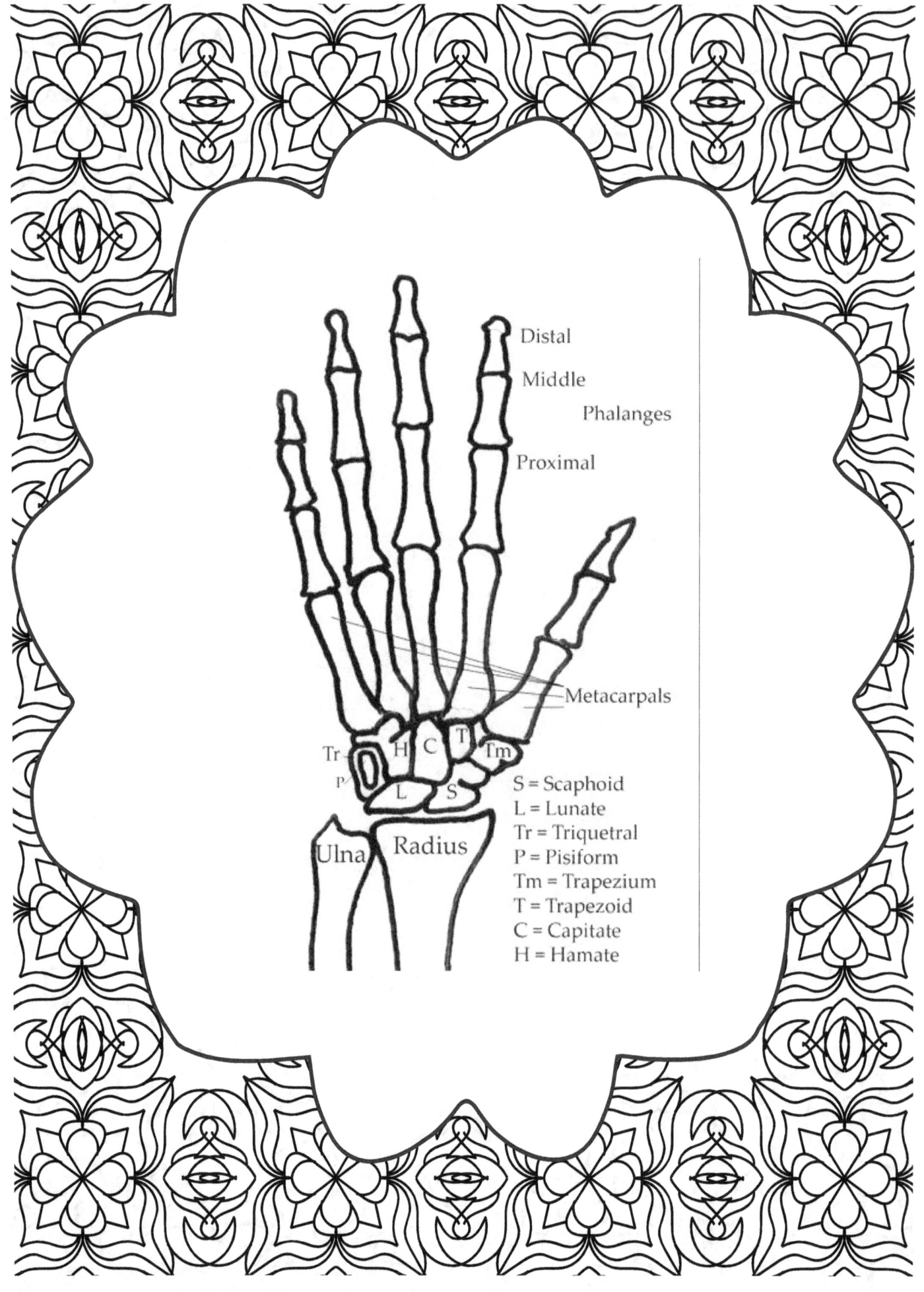

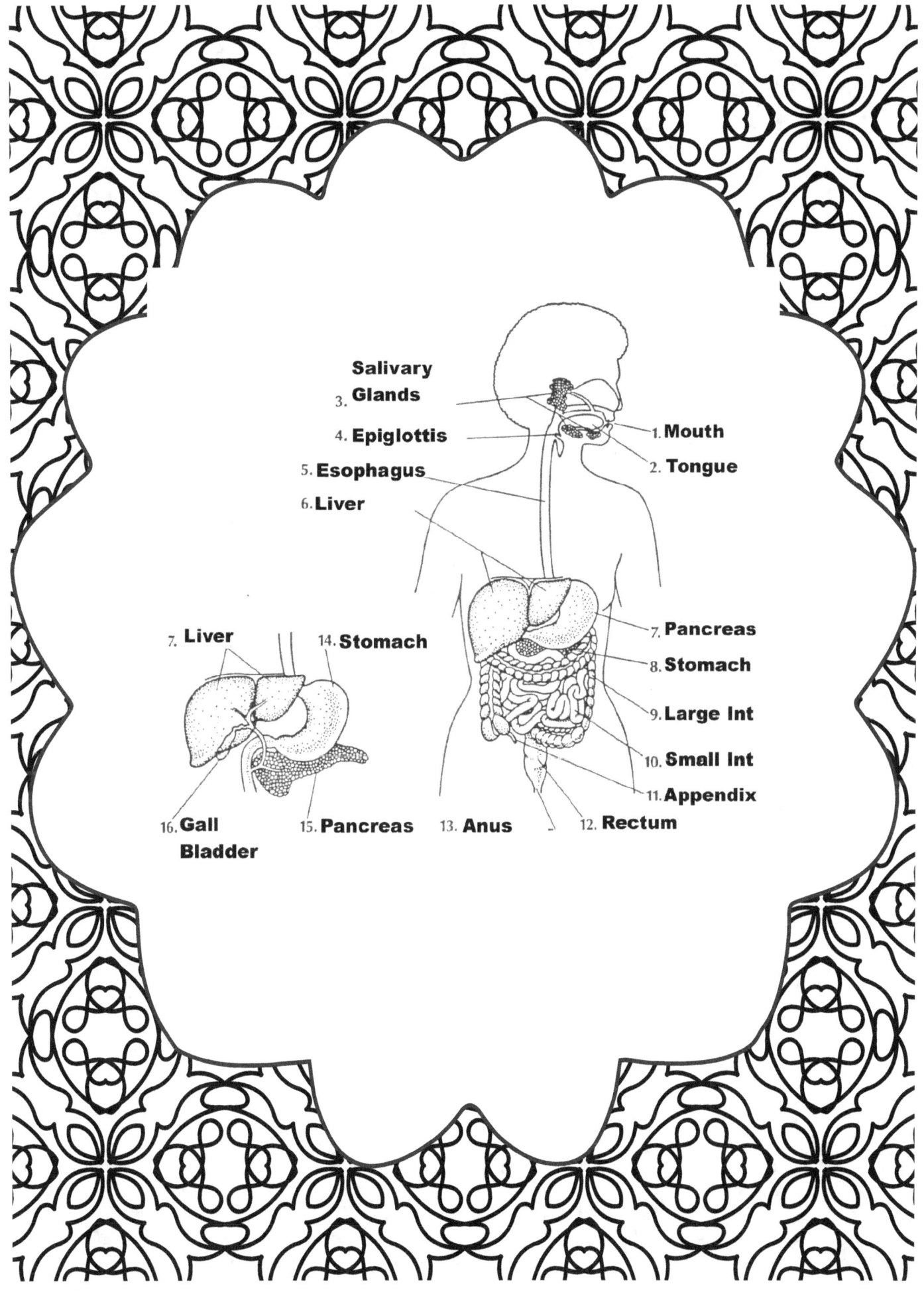

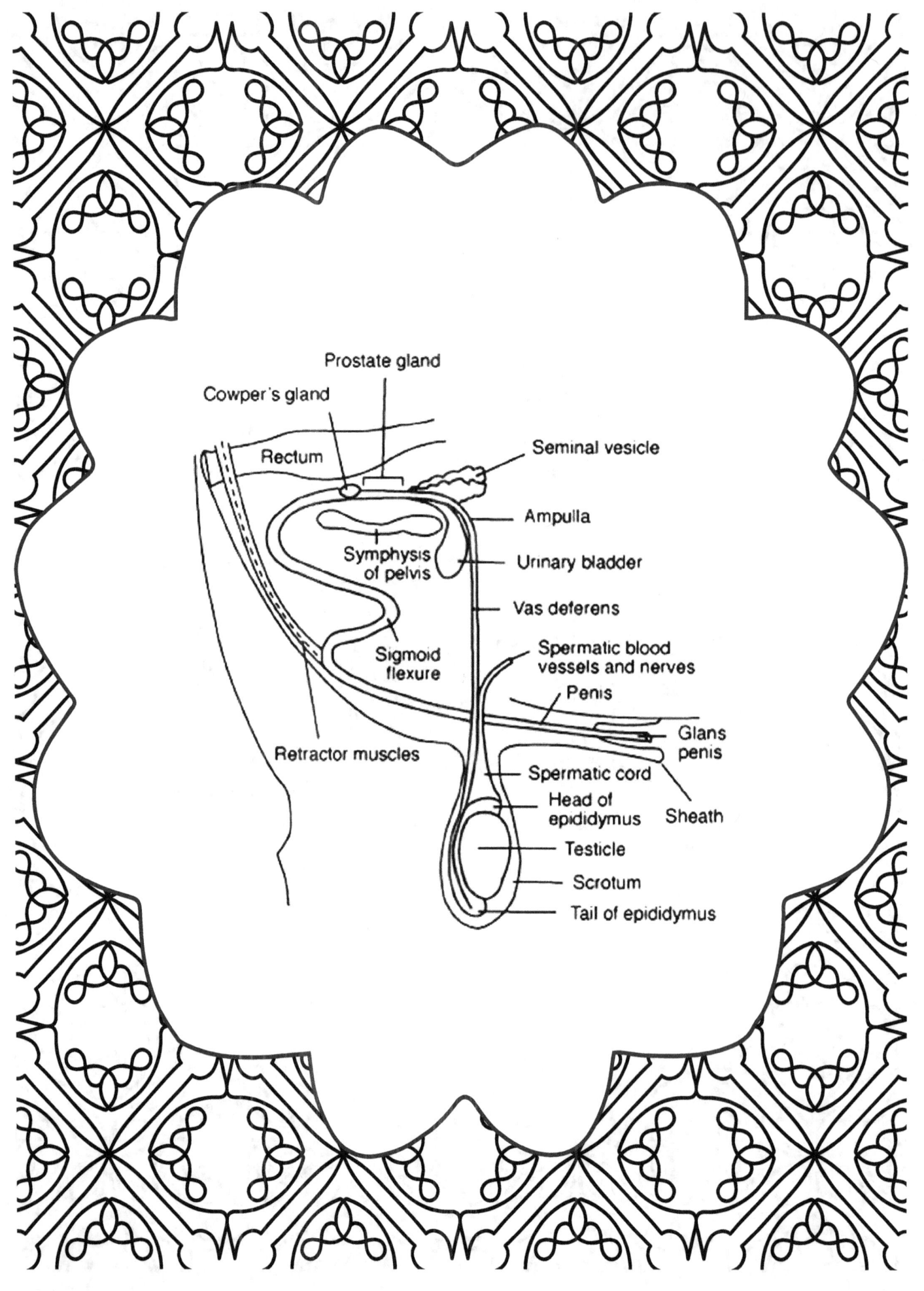

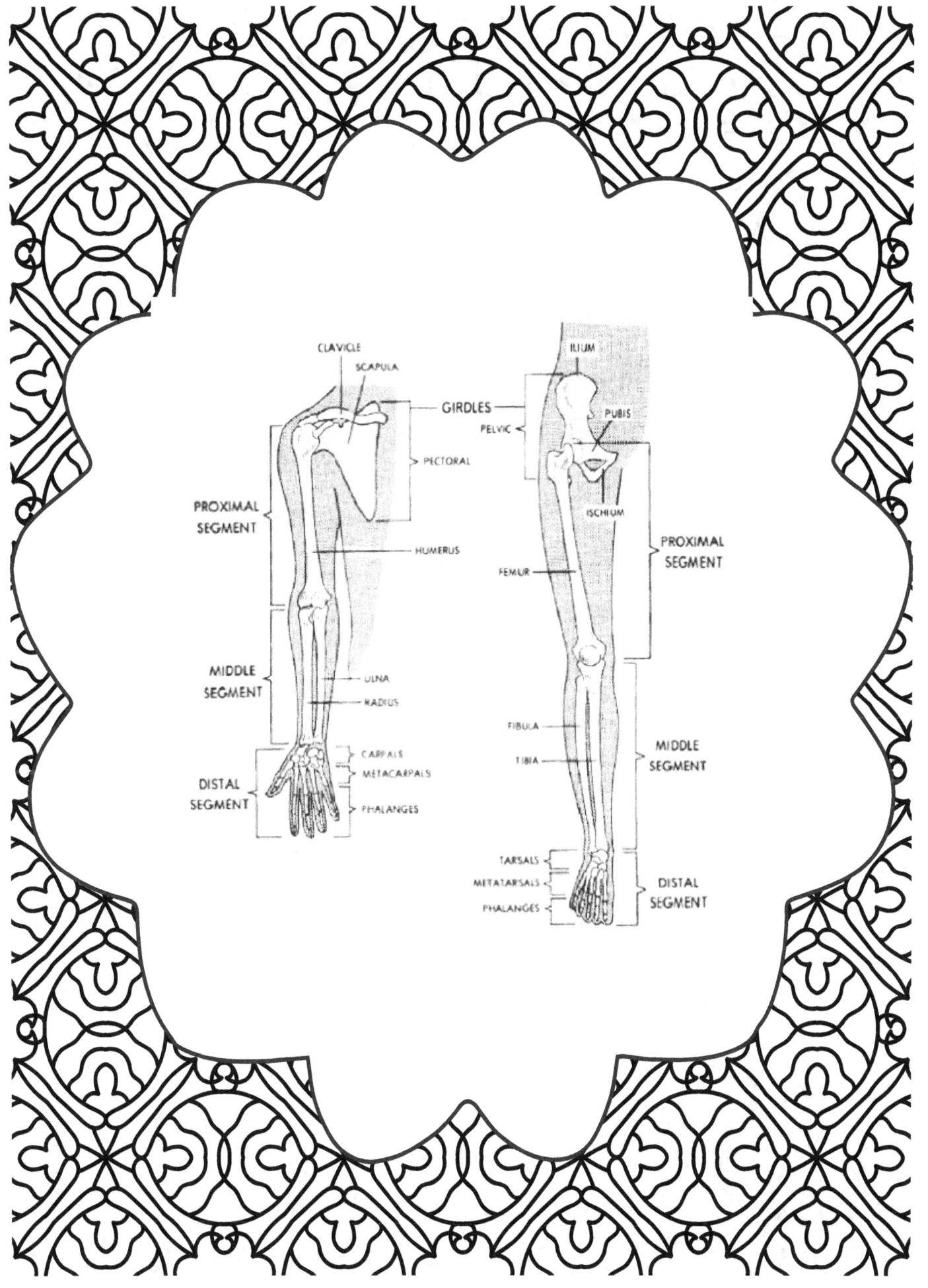

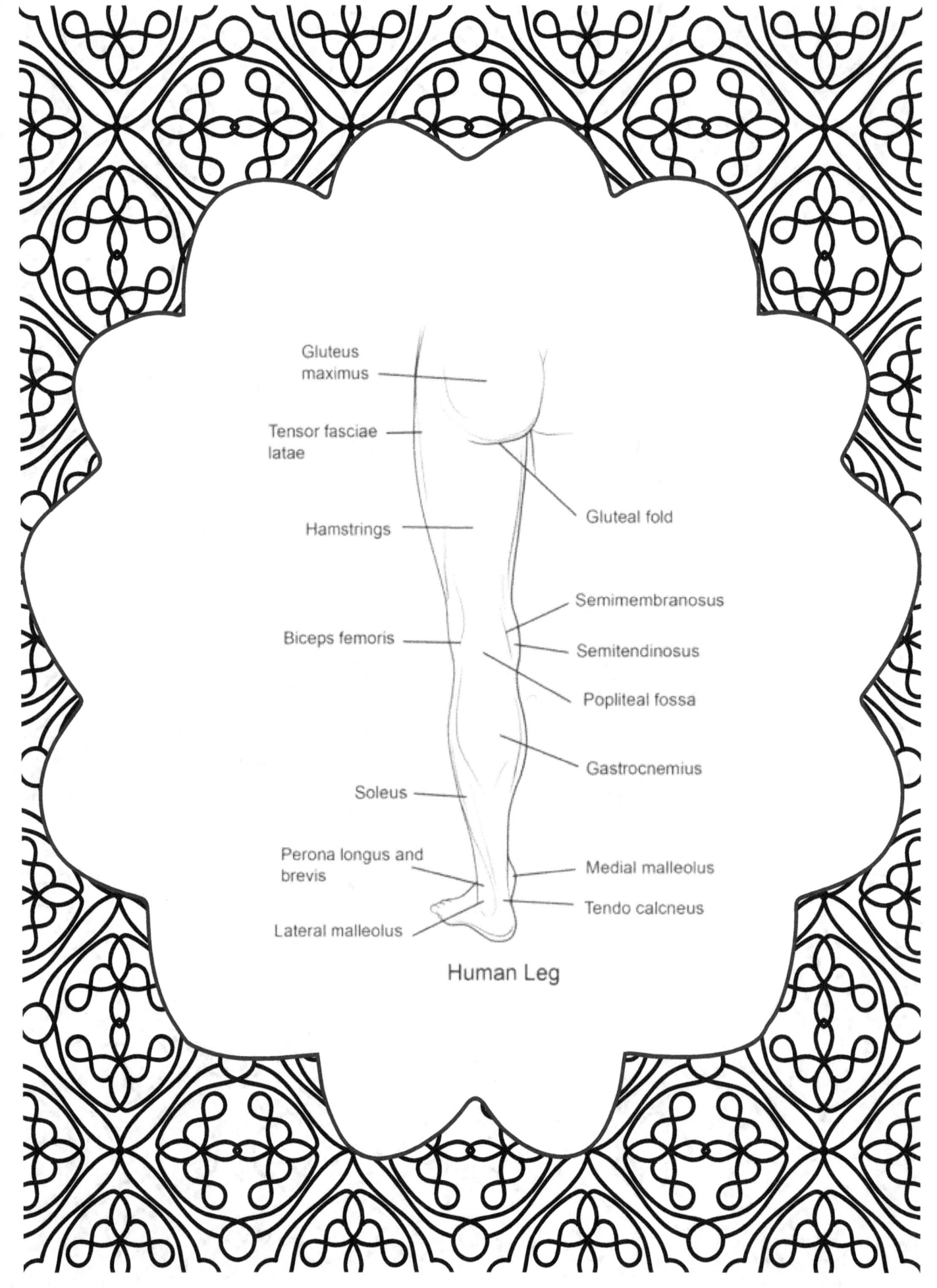

Gluteus maximus

Tensor fasciae latae

Hamstrings

Biceps femoris

Soleus

Perona longus and brevis

Lateral malleolus

Gluteal fold

Semimembranosus

Semitendinosus

Popliteal fossa

Gastrocnemius

Medial malleolus

Tendo calcneus

Human Leg

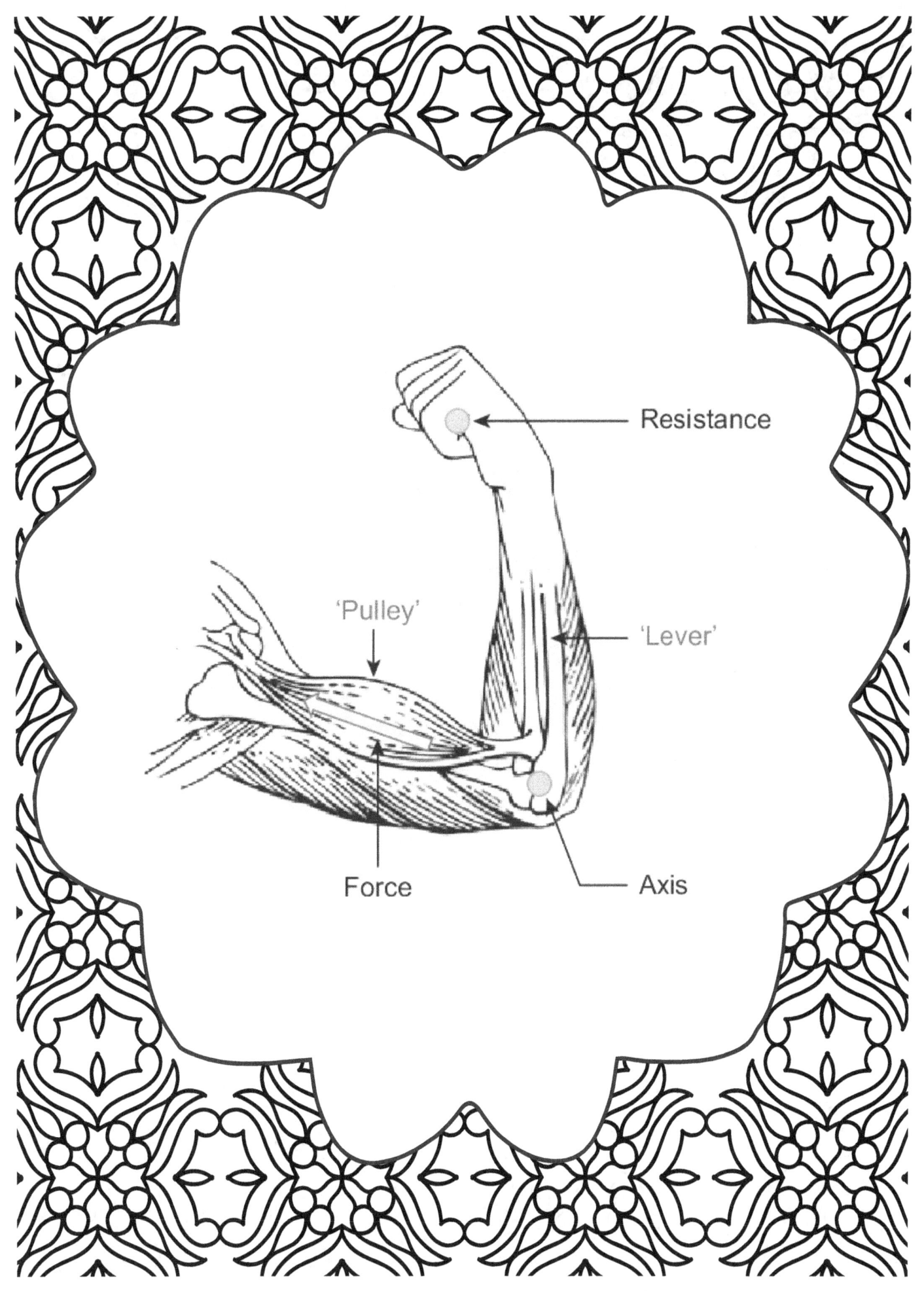

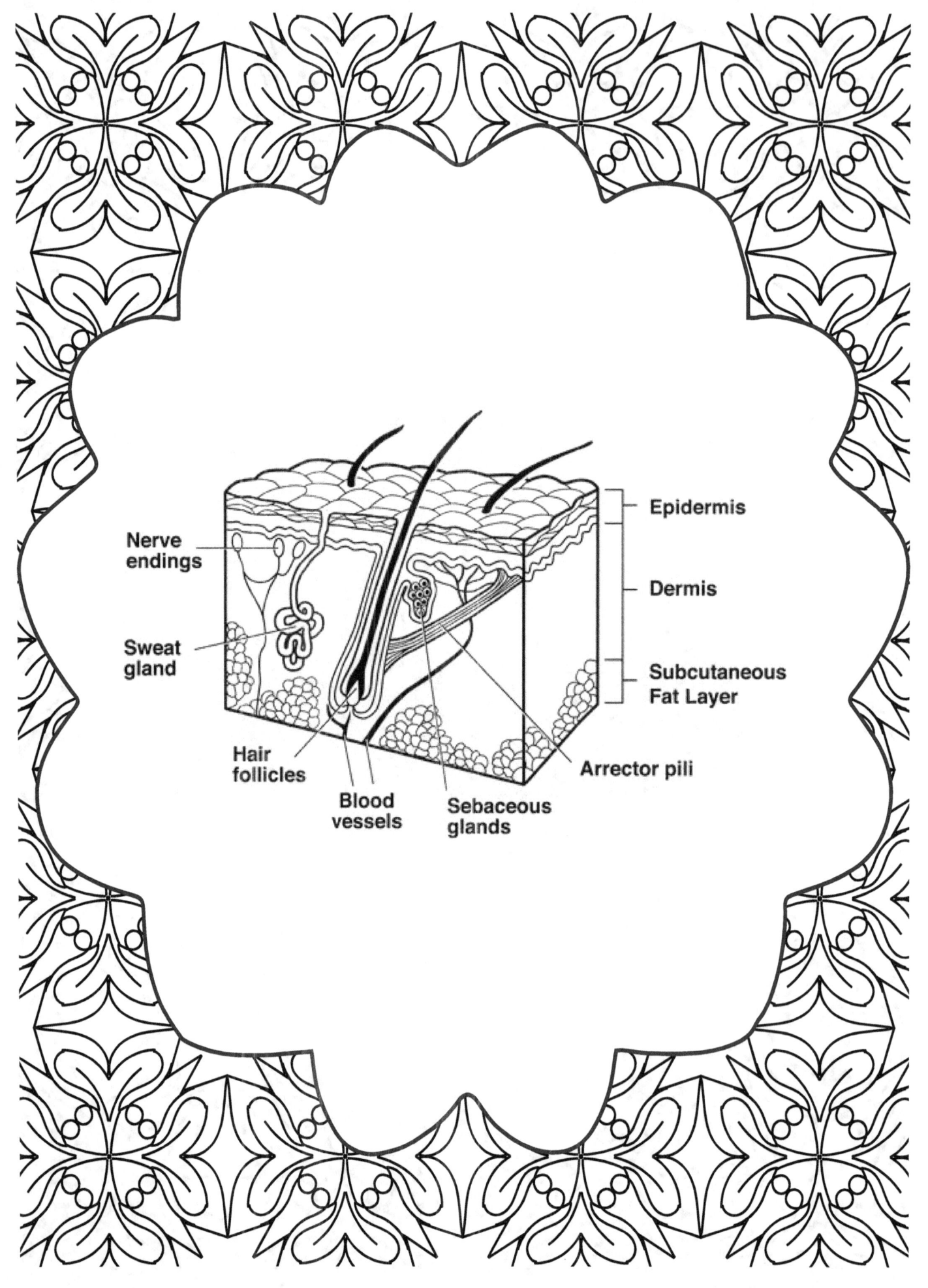

Nerve endings

Sweat gland

Hair follicles

Blood vessels

Sebaceous glands

Arrector pili

Epidermis

Dermis

Subcutaneous Fat Layer

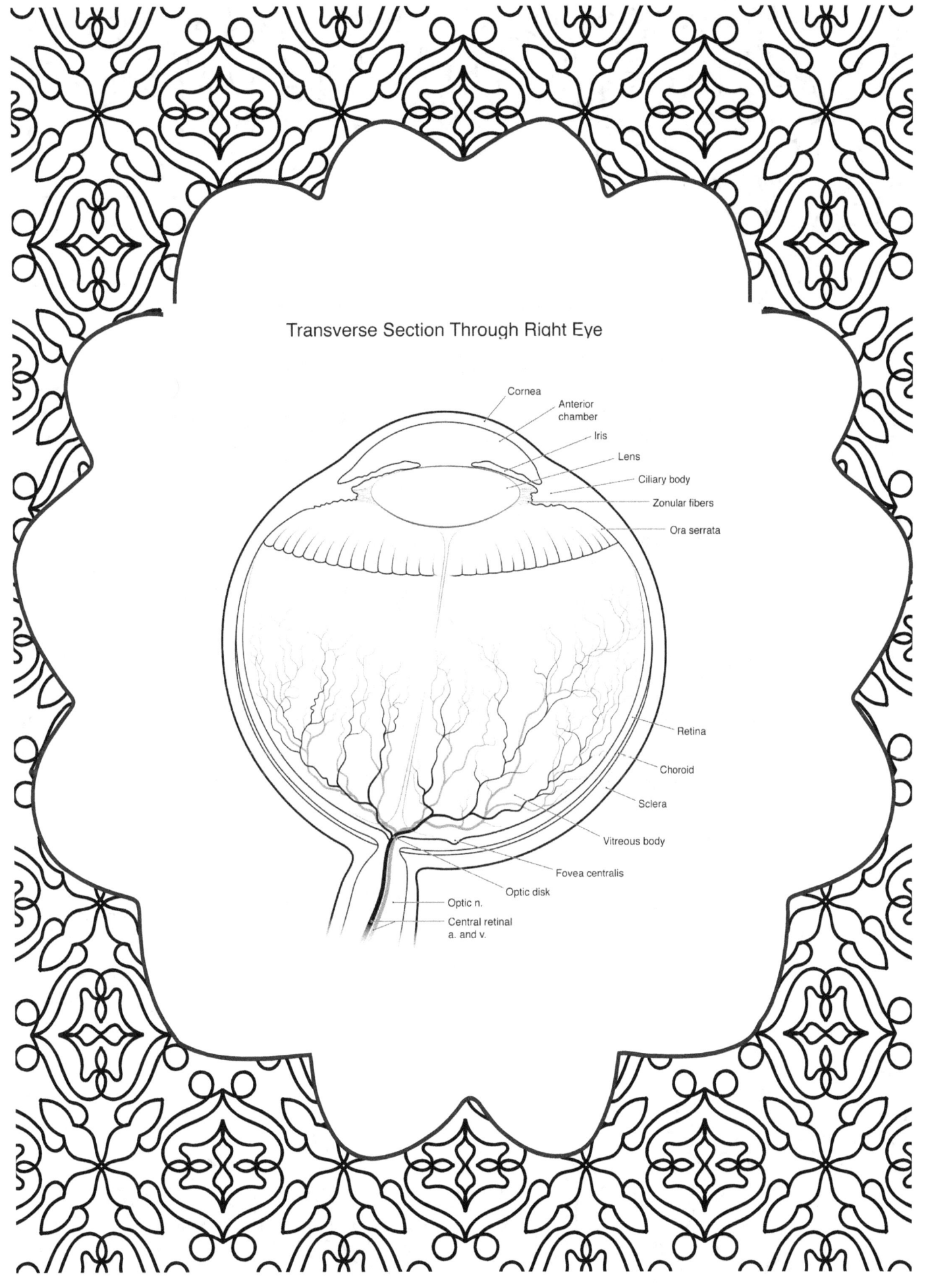

Transverse Section Through Right Eye

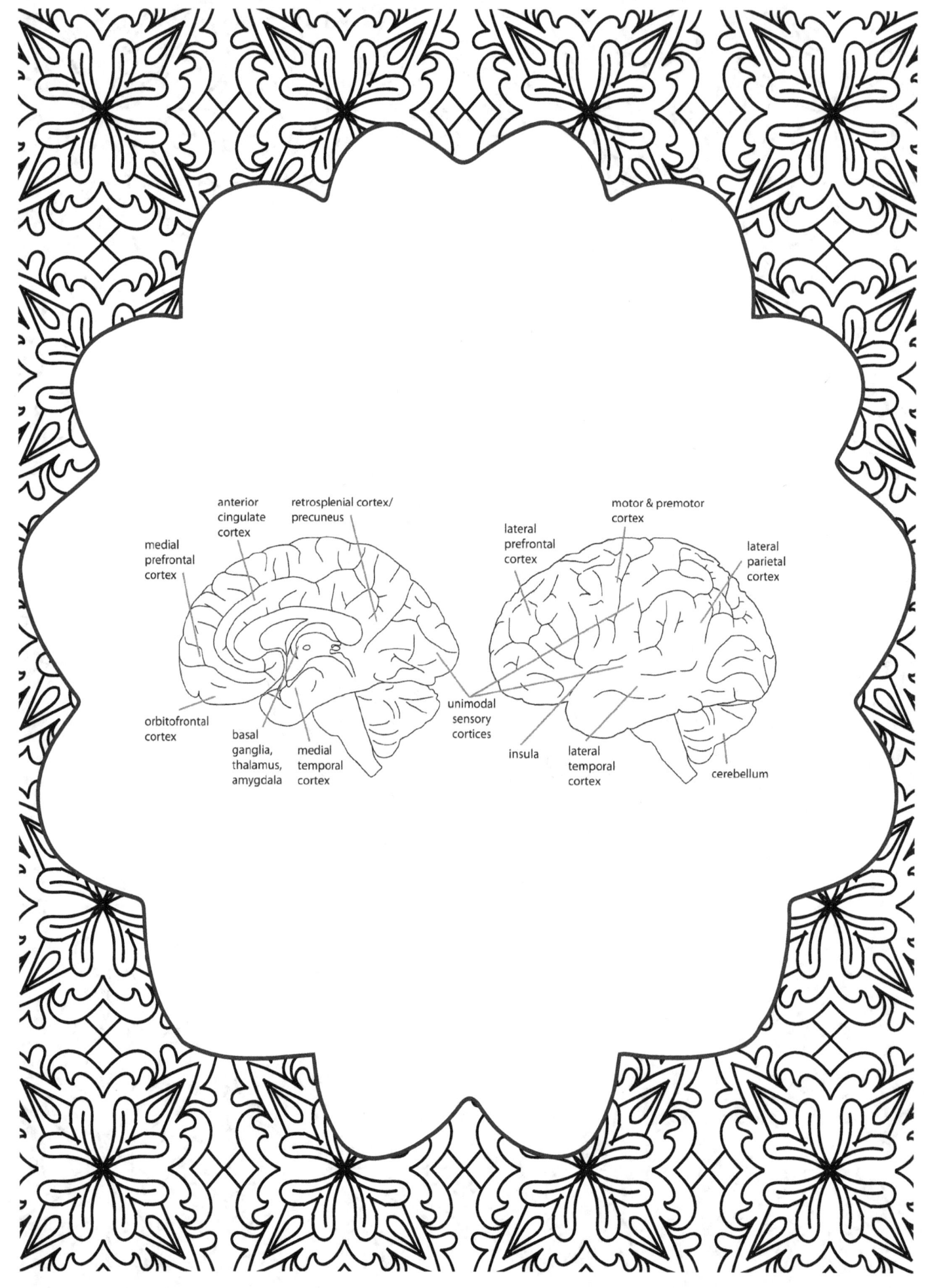